THE ROCKEFELLER UNIVERSITY

ACHIEVEMENTS

1901–2001

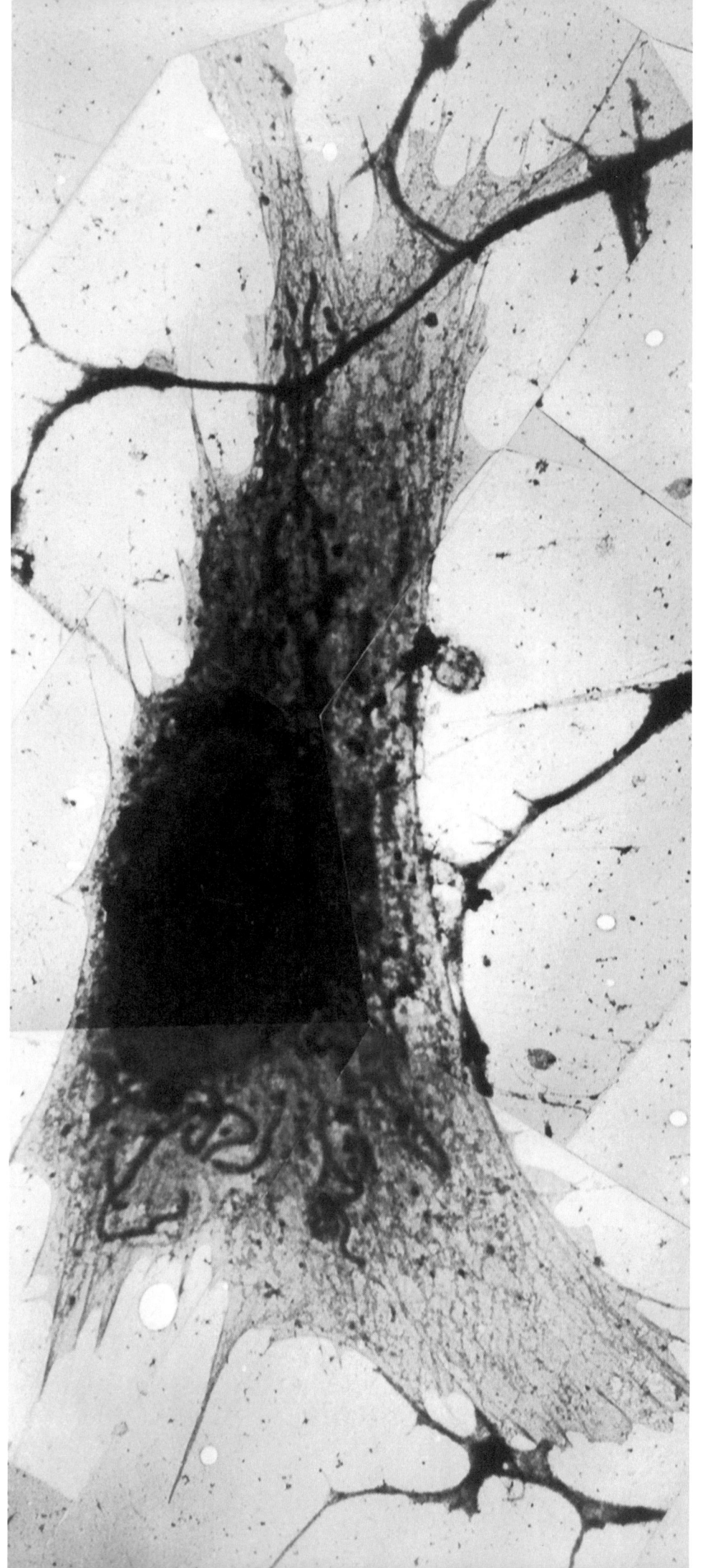

by Elizabeth Hanson

Introduction by Arnold J. Levine

Epilogue by David Rockefeller

THE ROCKEFELLER UNIVERSITY

ACHIEVEMENTS

A century of science for the benefit of humankind

1901–2001

© by The Rockefeller University Press 2000

All rights reserved

ISBN 0-87470-060-4

Printed in the United States of America

Frontispiece: The first electron micrograph of a whole cell, this composite of five images was published in 1945 by Keith Porter, Albert Claude, and Ernest Fullam.

Cover: Pneumococcus, the bacterium that Oswald Avery began investigating in 1913. Avery's work culminated in the discovery that DNA carries hereditary information, a finding that launched the era of molecular biology.

CONTENTS

Introduction
by Arnold J. Levine   7

FOUNDING
Part 1: The Rockefeller Institute for Medical Research   11

A VISION
Part 2: Medical Research Embraces the Physical Sciences   51

GROWTH
Part 3: From Institute to University   83

BIOLOGY, CHEMISTRY,
AND PHYSICS IN THE AGE
OF THE GENE
Part 4: Into the Future   115

Epilogue
by David Rockefeller   142

Endnotes   145

Acknowledgments   146

Faculty of The Rockefeller University   148

Index   151

Illustration Credits   154

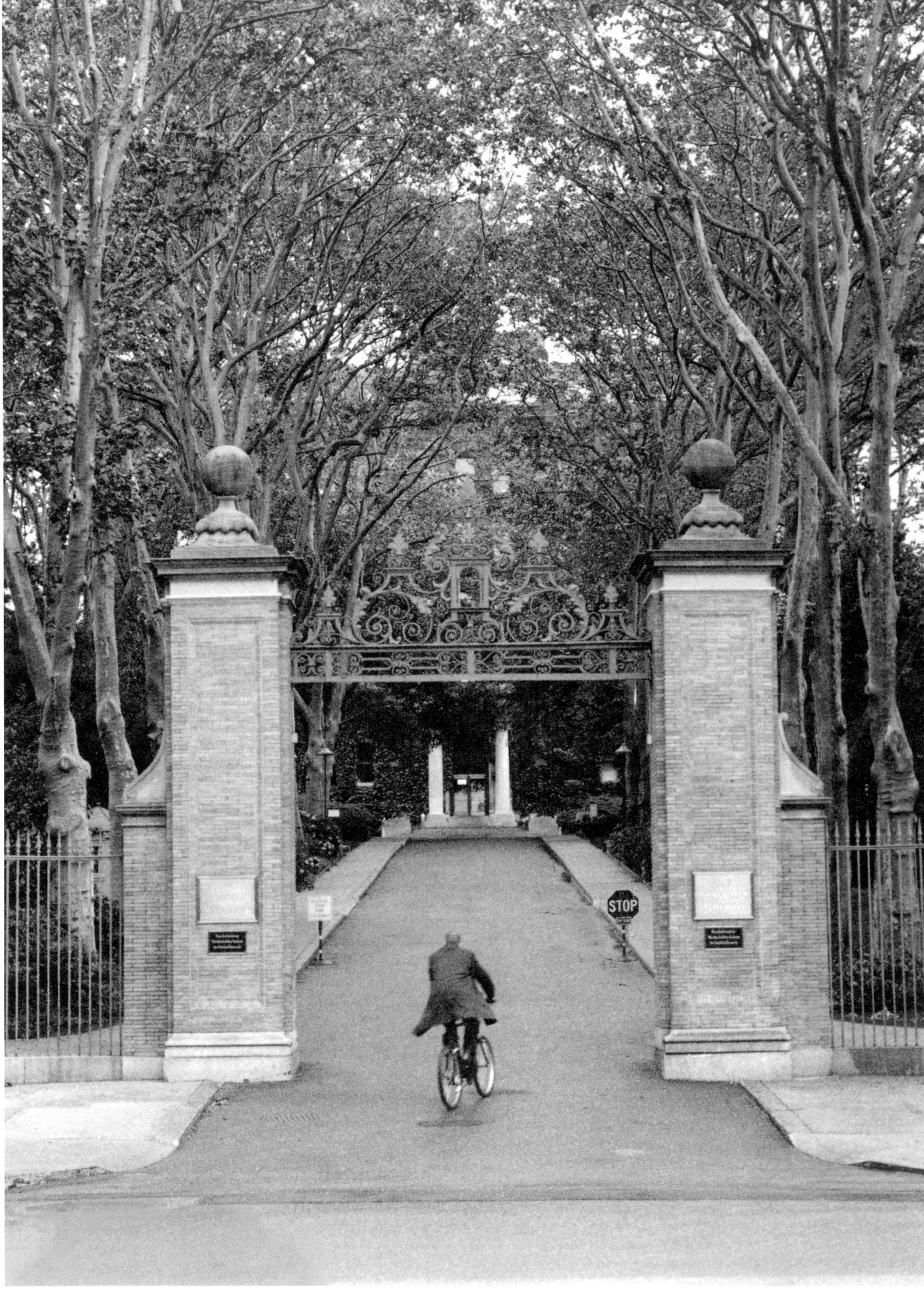

INTRODUCTION

by Arnold J. Levine, President

A century ago The Rockefeller Institute for Medical Research was incorporated. It was the idea of Frederick T. Gates, a layman who advised John D. Rockefeller on philanthropy and became convinced that scientific research would lead to cures for disease. This idea was revolutionary at a time when few medical schools offered students opportunities for research and no institution in the United States was devoted to studying the underlying causes of disease. Gates convinced Rockefeller to support a new research institute, and with a founding gift of $200,000 the first medical research institute in the United States was established.

This philanthropic gesture was far more important than the sum, which seems small by today's standards. With additional gifts from John D. Rockefeller, the Institute's budget in the first decades of the 20th century constituted nearly half of national expenditures on biomedical research. And from the beginning the scientific achievements of the Institute were correspondingly influential. The Institute's first director, Simon Flexner, assembled a stellar faculty. These outstanding researchers made The Rockefeller Institute, later renamed The Rockefeller University, the home of great events in science. Here Oswald Avery discovered that DNA carries hereditary information and the modern sciences of molecular and cell biology were born.

This small institution generated lines of research that have remained productive and important for a century. Peyton Rous, for example, found in 1911 that a virus can cause cancer. Subsequent studies with this virus led to the identification of the first cancer-causing gene. Such genes, called oncogenes, now form the basis for understanding the origins of cancer in humans. In between, Rous was awarded a Nobel Prize, and additional studies with this virus provided information that proved essential in fighting diseases like AIDS.

What made these early triumphs and the lasting success of the University possible? In part they resulted from John D. Rockefeller's long-term view of philanthropy coupled with the Institute's early devotion to basic research. Scientists were allowed to pursue their work without worry about quick payoffs. The founding Board of Directors maintained their faith that the unfettered pursuit of knowledge by the best minds would lead to important results.

The unique organization of the Institute also contributed to its productivity. With independent laboratories each reporting to the president, rather than departments as at universities, bureaucracy was kept to a minimum, lines of communication remained open, opportunities for collaborations abounded, and researchers had the flexibility to pursue the most compelling research problems.

Finally, the Institute's location in New York City—an international crossroads—made it a meeting place for scientists from around the world. Some stayed only long enough to learn new research techniques or collaborate on an experiment, whereas others remained for their entire careers. But always there has been a flow of ideas into the campus that has kept our approach to science fresh, and people who have worked at Rockefeller have gone on to contribute their knowledge and leadership to other institutions worldwide.

The mid-century transition from Institute to University formalized our long commitment to postgraduate education. It also validated Rockefeller's membership in the community of research universities dedicated to the pursuit of knowledge. Over the years our educational efforts have grown far beyond the University's campus. Through close mentoring of undergraduate and high school students, partnerships with educational and research institutions, public lectures, and other outreach efforts, we seek ways to contribute to the intellectual life of diverse communities and broaden public understanding of science.

Today The Rockefeller University is evolving a new culture on an old framework. This durable institutional structure allows us to remain intimate, flexible, and collaborative. We can adapt quickly to the changing currents of science while building on the groundwork laid by a century of discovery. Already our researchers are deeply engaged in a new era of science that is dominated by the study of genetics and genomics. Our singular history has brought us to the threshold of breakthroughs that will revolutionize the practice of medicine in the 21st century.

In this book we pay tribute to the accomplishments of our past and describe the research of today. As we celebrate the centennial of The Rockefeller University we want to remind both the Rockefeller community and the world beyond of the remarkable achievements of our scientists and the continuity of our ideals. While acknowledging the past we are looking ahead. The years to come promise equally significant successes—advances in research driven by our continued dedication to science for the improvement of health and life.

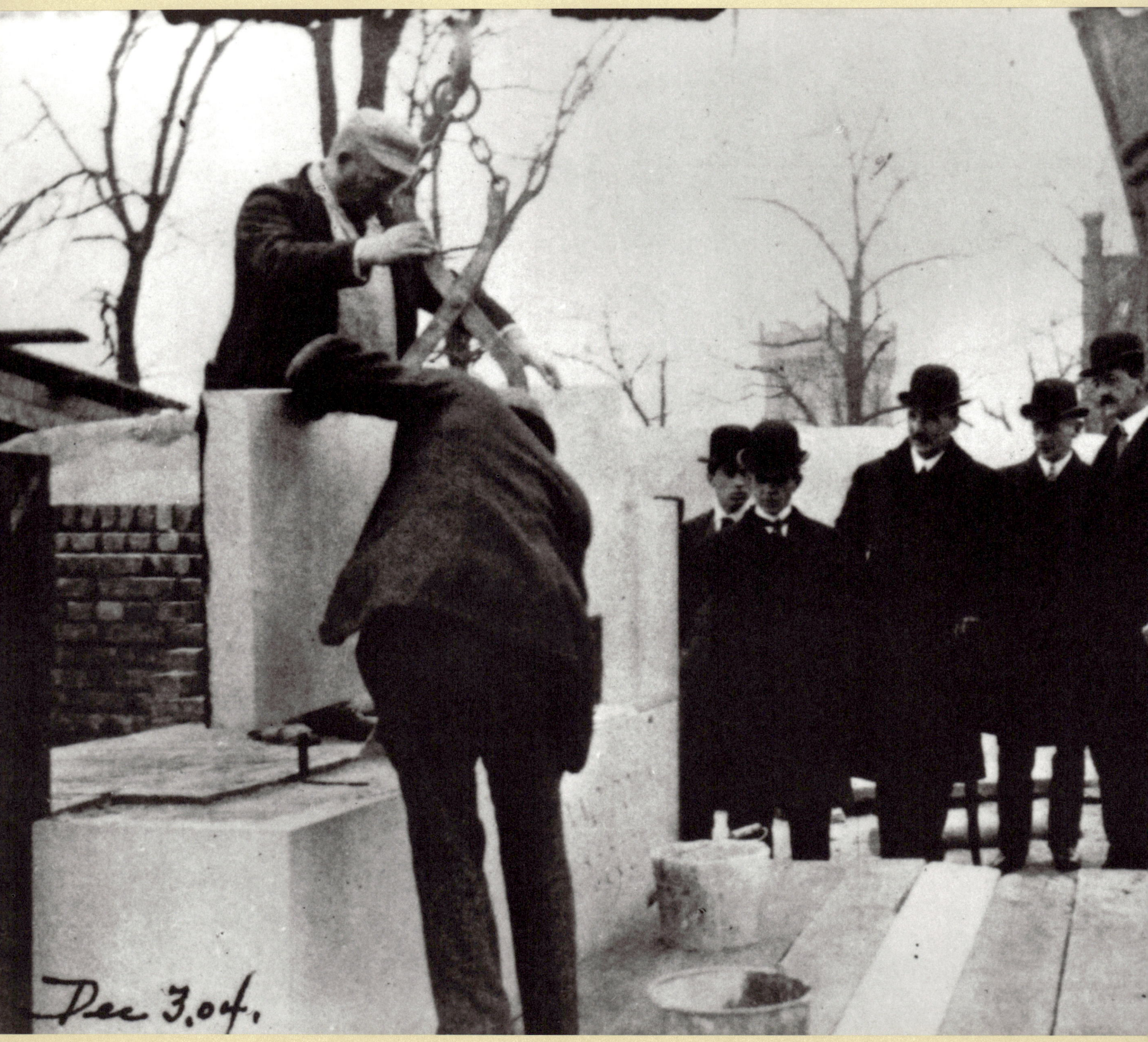

The cornerstone of Founder's Hall was laid December 3, 1904. Looking on in the background are members of the Board of Directors (from left to right): L. Emmett Holt, Hermann M. Biggs, Simon Flexner, and T. Mitchell Prudden.

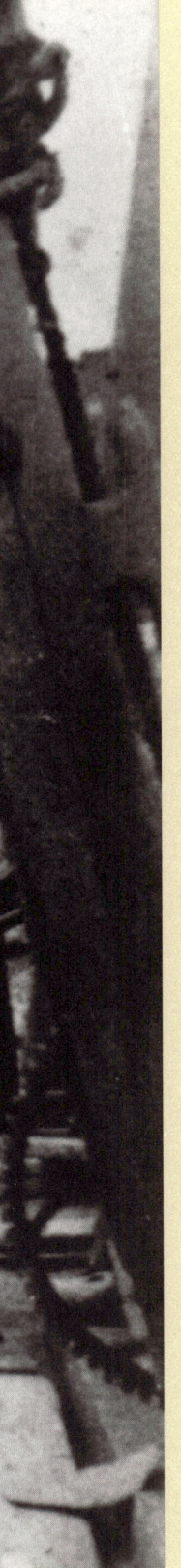

FOUNDING

Part 1: The Rockefeller Institute for Medical Research

The leading causes of death at the turn of the 20th century were infectious diseases. Pneumonia, influenza, diphtheria, and typhoid fever were fearsome threats, and in the United States tuberculosis alone caused as many as one in four deaths. A century later, few Americans die from these illnesses, and the dread they once evoked is lost to history. Doctors of the day, however, could do little to combat them. "Pneumonia," reported the leading medical textbook of the day, "is a self-limited disease, which can neither be aborted nor cut short by any known means at our command." For most illness the recommended therapy consisted of "good nursing and careful diet." The need for new ways to understand and treat disease was urgent.

In 1897 John D. Rockefeller's chief advisor on philanthropy, Frederick T. Gates, brought this state of affairs to Rockefeller's attention. In his earlier career as a Baptist minister Gates had the opportunity to talk with a wide range of medical practitioners in his congregation—not only physicians, but homeopaths, Christian Scientists, and faith healers as well. The most intelligent and the best educated of them admitted that medical science had a cure for perhaps one in a hundred patients, prompting Gates to conclude that "medicine as generally taught and practiced in the United States was practically futile." Gates determined to find out for himself "what really lay in the minds of doctors in active practice." During a two-month vacation he pored over the textbook *Principles and Practice of Medicine* by the eminent physician William Osler. He found that Osler was an expert at describing disease symptoms and making diagnoses. But "[t]o a layman like me, demanding cures, he had no word of comfort whatever," wrote Gates. With his suspicions about medicine's powerlessness confirmed, Gates submitted an "earnest" memo to John D. Rockefeller that set in motion the founding of The Rockefeller Institute for Medical Research.

"It became clear to me that medicine could hardly hope to become a science until medicine was endowed, and qualified men were enabled to give themselves to uninterrupted study and investigation, on ample salary, entirely independent of practice," Gates later recalled. "To this end, it seemed to me an institute of medical research ought to be established in the United States."

Gates' conviction that scientific research could lay the groundwork for curing disease was both unusual and farsighted, and his proposal was timely. In the late 19th century European researchers were bringing the tools of the laboratory to bear on problems of human health. In France, Louis Pasteur promoted the germ theory of disease, debunking the long-held notion that rotting material generated germs spontaneously, and theories that miasmas—essentially bad air, or vapors—caused illness. In Germany, Robert Koch and his students discovered the bacteria that cause tuberculosis, cholera, anthrax, and other diseases. Yet, although this new knowledge held out promise for finding cures, at the turn of the century it had little impact on the practice of medicine. In the United States, there was no place devoted exclusively to medical research.

Gates' proposal to fund a biomedical research institute intrigued Rockefeller. As always in matters of philanthropy, Rockefeller proceeded cautiously. He favored projects that were likely both to succeed and to benefit many people. Since suffering from disease was a universal scourge, medical science seemed an appropriate endeavor to support. Its results would aid people around the world. Still, there were practical matters to consider. Would the new research center be affiliated with an existing university or medical school, or would it be independent? In what city should it be located? Given the embryonic state of medical research in 1897, it was not even clear whether enough qualified scientists could be found to staff a research institute, or whether its need was adequately recognized in the medical profession. A few years earlier, the University of Chicago had attempted to persuade Rockefeller to finance a medical school, but negotiations broke down when the university resisted Rockefeller's demand for a department devoted to research rather than teaching.

Furthermore, there were philosophical hurdles. Rockefeller and Gates considered affiliating the new institute with Harvard and Columbia Universities, both of which had medical schools. Distinguished as those universities were, even they were tarred

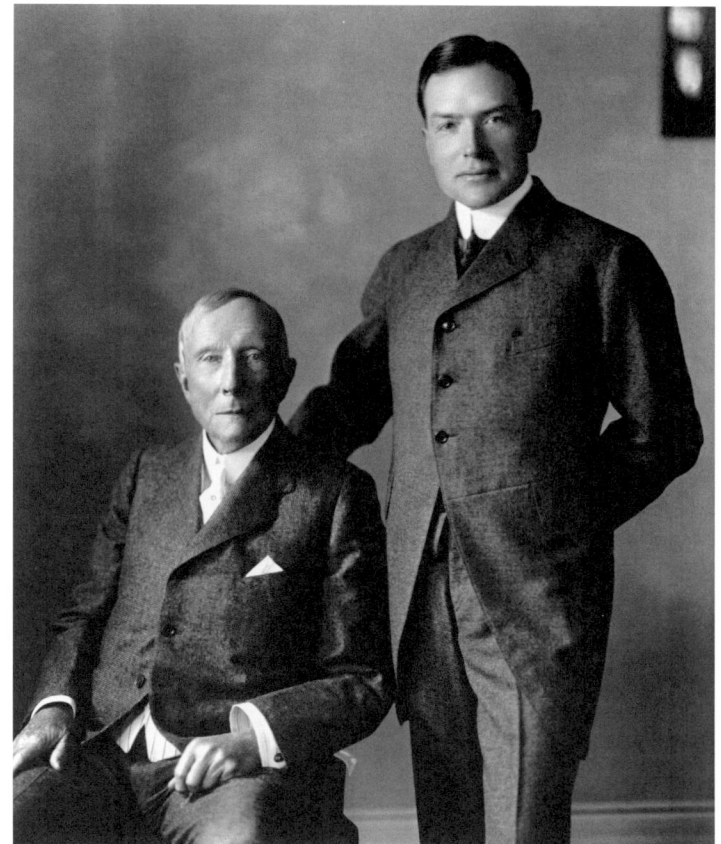

The Institute was founded through the philanthropy of John D. Rockefeller (seated) and the leadership of his son John D. Rockefeller Jr. (standing). (c. 1914)

by the low esteem in which medical education was held at the turn of the century. Students with little more than a high school education enrolled at hundreds of proprietary medical schools where instructors depended directly on student fees for their livelihood. To make things more complicated, association with a medical school would imply endorsement of one of two approaches to medical practice. The allopathic majority often advocated active interventions like surgery, agents to induce vomiting, and even bleeding. The homeopathic minority promoted gentler methods of healing. Rockefeller himself consulted a homeopath. Gates found both camps hopelessly unscientific.

John D. Rockefeller consulted with his son, John D. Rockefeller Jr., his aide in affairs of philanthropy, and came to the conclusion that an independent institute for medical research would bring the most benefit to humanity. Unlike university faculty, researchers at an independent institute would not be burdened with teaching and administrative duties—they could devote all their efforts to research. And an independent institute could remain aloof from the allopath-homeopath debate. It would be a place for disinterested inquiry into the science underlying health and disease. Furthermore, the institute would be in New York City, which was Rockefeller's home and headquarters of the Standard Oil Company.

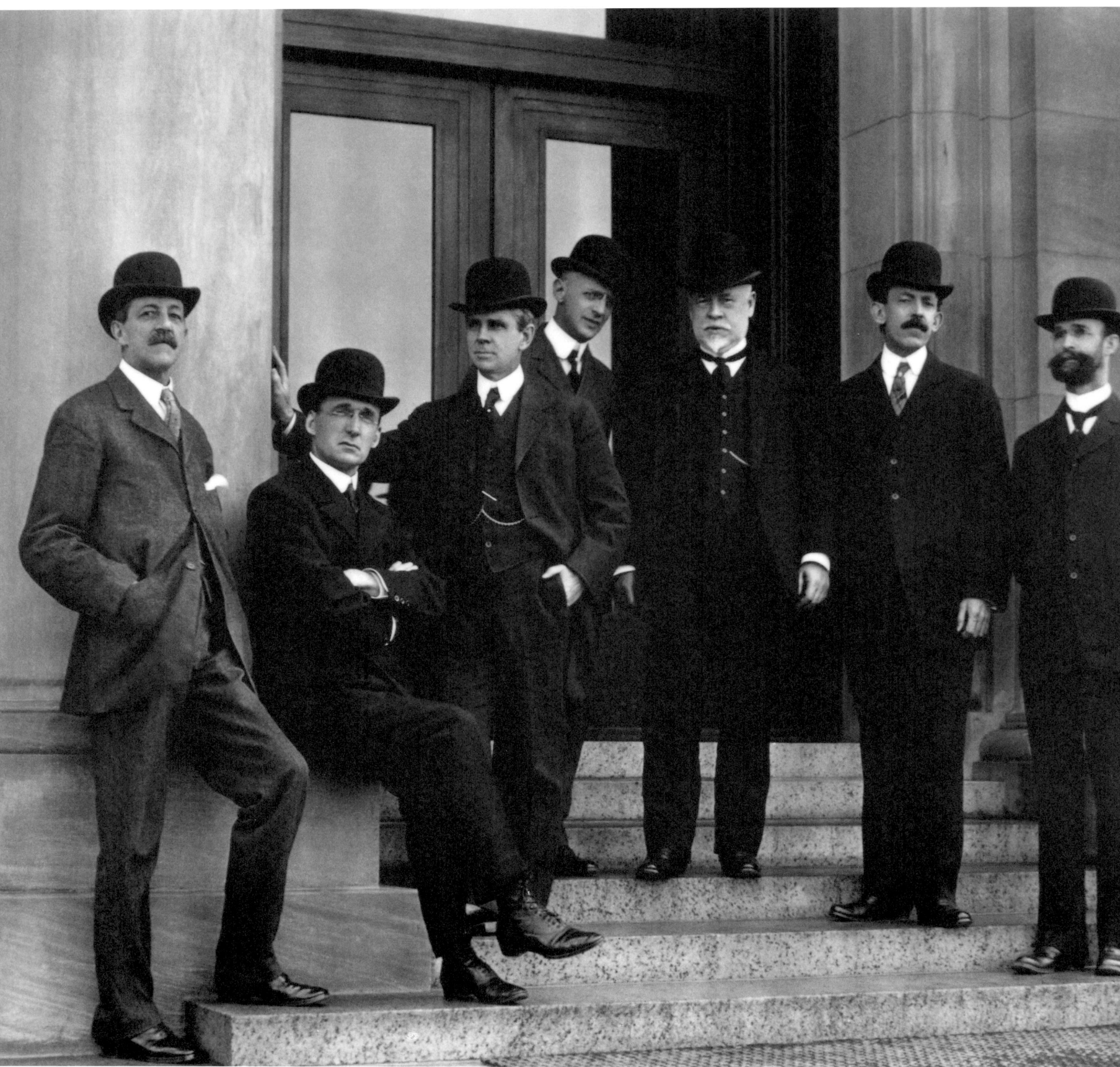

The first Board of Directors of The Rockefeller Institute for Medical Research poses on the steps of Founder's Hall in 1909. From left to right: T. Mitchell Prudden, Christian A. Herter, L. Emmett Holt, Simon Flexner, William H. Welch, Hermann M. Biggs, and Theobald Smith.

John D. Rockefeller Jr. gathered information about medical research and the advisability of investing in it. A typically positive opinion came from William H. Welch, founding dean of the Johns Hopkins University Medical School, one of the few medical schools equipped with research laboratories at the time. "I am confident that the establishment in this country of a properly endowed institute on the general lines of the French Pasteur Institute would be of the greatest benefit to medical science and to humanity," he wrote. "I know of no other way in which the expenditure of a like sum of money would be expected to yield greater returns in the advancement of useful knowledge and of the physical well-being of mankind."

Personal tragedy helped decide the issue. In December 1900 Rockefeller's first grandchild, three-year-old John Rockefeller McCormick, became ill with scarlet fever. He died on January 2, 1901, a heartbreaking reminder of how ill-equipped the medical profession was to deal with infectious diseases. The best physicians available could offer no remedy.

Within months Rockefeller Jr. met with the prominent pediatrician Emmett Holt, who was also his fellow parishioner at the Fifth Avenue Baptist Church, and Christian Herter, a physician known for the research he conducted in a small laboratory in his home. Rockefeller Jr. asked Holt and Herter to assemble a Board of Directors. Turning to William Welch for advice, they added four more members, all physicians. Welch became the first chairman of the Board—a position he held until his death in 1933.

By the end of April 1901 Rockefeller had pledged a sum of $200,000 to the planned Institute, to be allocated over a period of 10 years. Soon after, the Board met to adopt bylaws, and on June 14, 1901, The Rockefeller Institute for Medical Research was incorporated. Rather than building a facility, the Board used Rockefeller's donation to provide grants and fellowships to researchers in existing laboratories. Like the scientists he supported, Rockefeller undertook an experiment; before committing funds to a permanent Institute, he aimed to discover whether the project would be worthwhile.

The 1901-1902 report of the Institute's activities announced optimistically that "conditions are now not only favorable but urgent for such expansion of the scope of the Institute as will enable it adequately to cover the field so full of promise of the highest usefulness." This confidence and the success of the first year's grant recipients

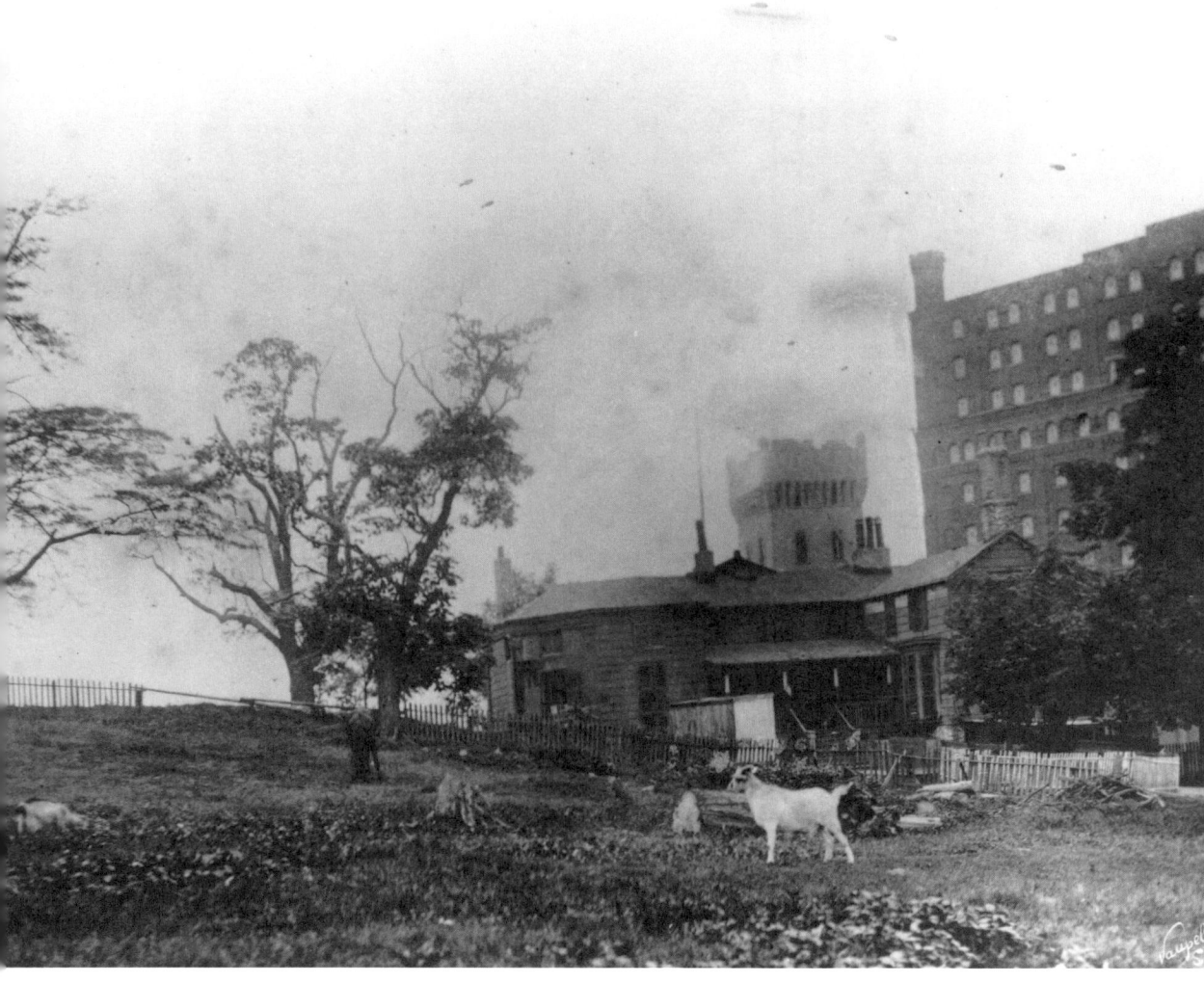

The former Schermerhorn farm became the site of The Rockefeller Institute in 1903.

must have convinced John D. Rockefeller that his experiment would prove successful, for in 1902 he altered his original philanthropic plan and pledged $1 million to the Institute.

In 1903 the Institute, which was renting temporary laboratory space in a building at 50th Street and Lexington Avenue, used some of this money to purchase property for a permanent home: 13 acres of land on the East River between 64th and 68th Streets, the last open tract in a neighborhood of tenements and breweries. Formerly the Schermerhorn farm, it was still grazed by a few goats. Researchers moved into the Institute's first building in 1906. Now called Founder's Hall, it was a modest structure perched on a bluff overlooking the East River. This outpost for research at the edge of the city would quickly become a hub for international scientific exchange.

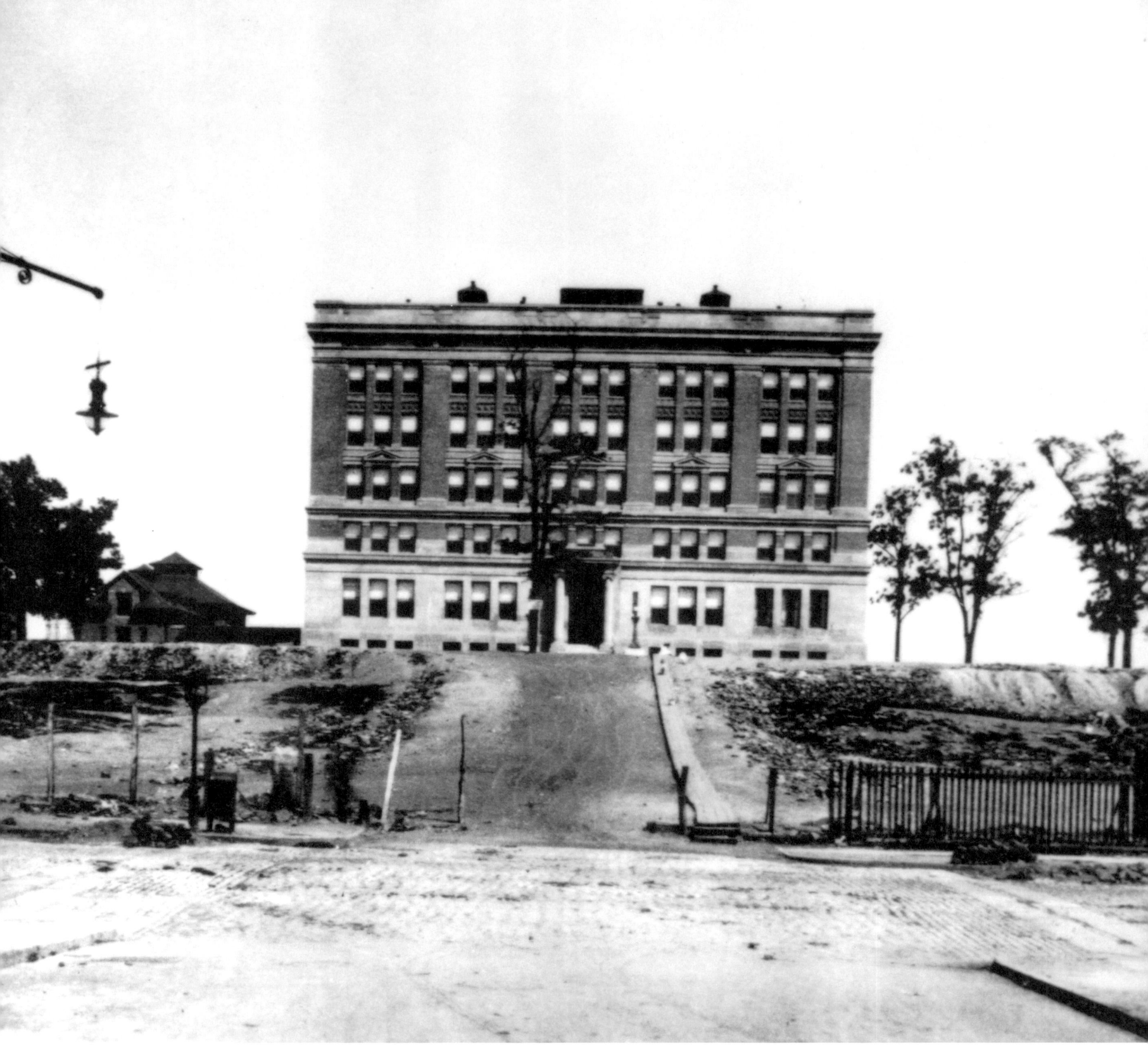

Founder's Hall, completed in 1906, housed the Institute's first permanent laboratories.

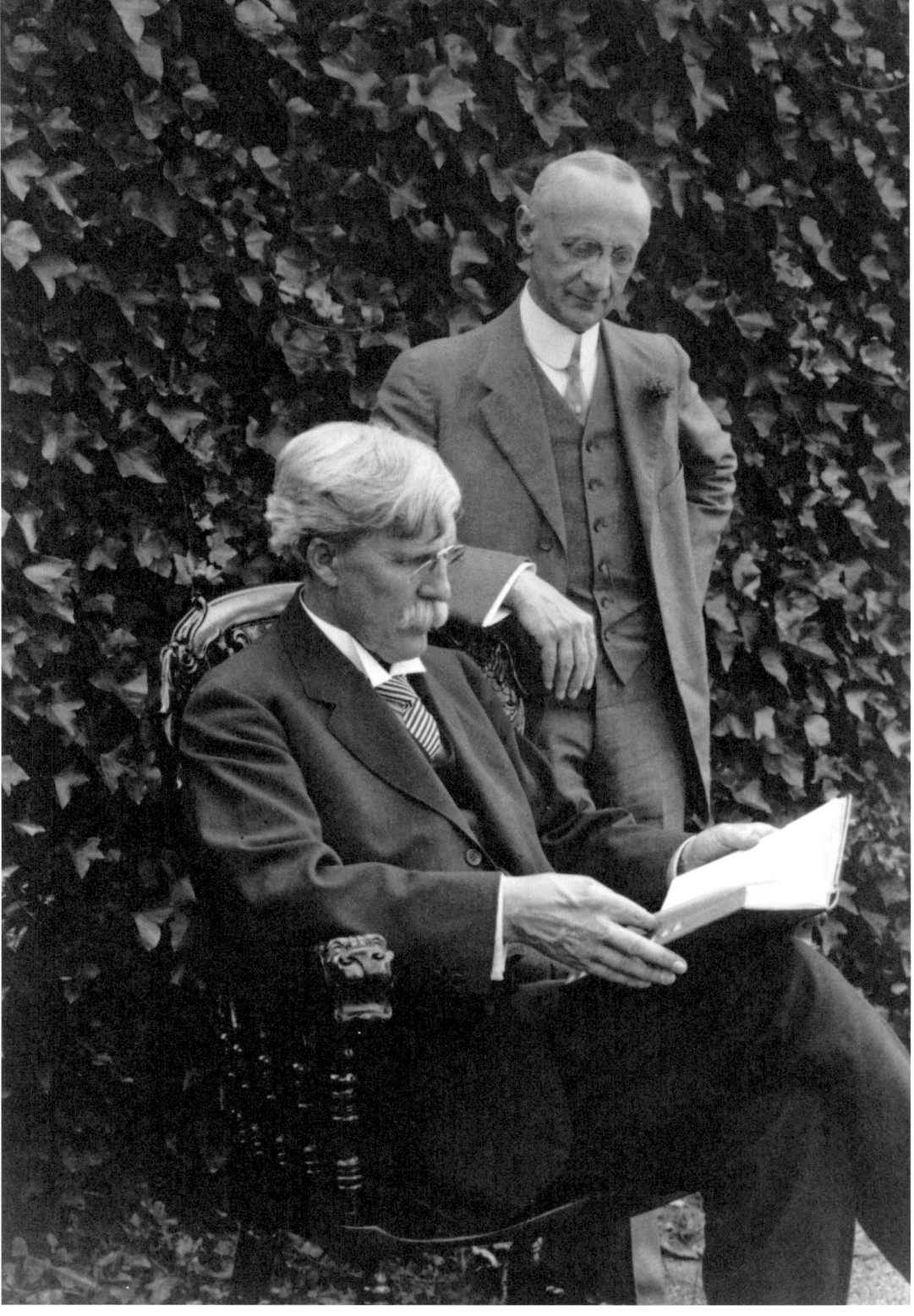

Frederick T. Gates was John D. Rockefeller's chief advisor on philanthropy (seated); Simon Flexner served as the Institute's first director (standing).

Simon Flexner's Vision

In the Institute's first year the Board of Directors oversaw its work, but a permanent director was needed. The top two candidates were already members of the Board. Theobald Smith refused the job. Well-established as chair of comparative pathology at Harvard University and renowned for his discovery that Texas cattle fever was transmitted by a tick, Smith was unwilling to assume the risk of heading a new and uncertain enterprise. Next in line was a younger man, Simon Flexner, not yet 40, who had been a protégé of William Welch at Johns Hopkins.

In 1902, when the Board asked Flexner to head the fledgling Rockefeller Institute for Medical Research, he was a newly appointed professor of pathology at the University of Pennsylvania and gaining national recognition. He had a reputation as a microbe hunter, having traveled to the Philippines in 1899 to study health conditions in the newly acquired U.S. territory, where he discovered a bacterium that causes dysentery. When plague broke out in 1901 in San Francisco, the federal government sent Flexner there to make recommendations for eradicating the disease. In his position at Penn, Flexner would have had the opportunity to build a world-class pathology department. It was not an appointment to give up lightly.

Welch and the other Board members convinced Flexner that the new Institute in New York presented the chance for an even more brilliant career—never mind that it was unendowed and without staff or physical facilities. Flexner wrote to the Board outlining the terms under which he would accept the post, including a detailed plan for expanding the grant-giving committee to a brick-and-mortar institution. The Board endorsed Flexner's proposal and made him director of the Institute in 1902. The vision Flexner articulated and carried out over the next three decades would shape The Rockefeller Institute's beginnings and leave a lasting legacy.

Flexner proposed that the Institute's work should "cover the entire field of medical research." More than bacteriology and pathology, it should also encompass chemistry and any other science that could be brought to bear on the problems of human disease. Flexner's idea—unique at the time—was to organize the Institute around a number of laboratories, each headed by an independent investigator. Flexner's departure from convention went further still. Unlike a university science faculty, this would have no departments. Nor would researchers be hired to fit predetermined specialties; instead, Flexner sought the most creative minds in medical research and set them free to pursue problems of their own choosing. The Institute's role, he said, was to support them with salaries, facilities, and the necessary assistants and technicians.

In so saying, Flexner staked the success of the Institute on his ability to hire exceptional people. "I am convinced that there is just one way to keep up and not go backwards," Flexner wrote, "and that lies in trying for the best man, who may decline to come, rather than go for men less good, who you know will accept your invitation." Indeed, many of the "best men" turned Flexner down. The Institute had no guarantee of permanence. Scientists in the secure and familiar fold of academia would have to be persuaded to leave. Moreover, the idea of pursuing research full-time was then so novel as to seem almost bizarre. Jacques Loeb, the renowned physiologist who came to Rockefeller in 1910, later remarked that he had doubted whether he could fill his days with it.

But Flexner had a keen eye for scientific talent. He was always on the watch for exceptional researchers, and he found ways to nurture the development of young scientists. Among the first investigators Flexner brought to the Institute were Samuel Meltzer, who gave up a successful medical practice for the opportunity to pursue his research in experimental physiology full-time, and P.A.T. Levene, who became the foremost nucleic acid chemist of the early 20th century. Flexner set up a laboratory for himself as well, to continue his investigations on human infectious diseases. He hired Eugene Opie to work with him, and he brought Hideyo Noguchi from his University of Pennsylvania laboratory. In 1906, when the permanent laboratory building opened, Alexis Carrel joined the staff, starting a laboratory for experimental surgery. Carrel received a Nobel Prize in 1912 for his achievements in suturing blood vessels.

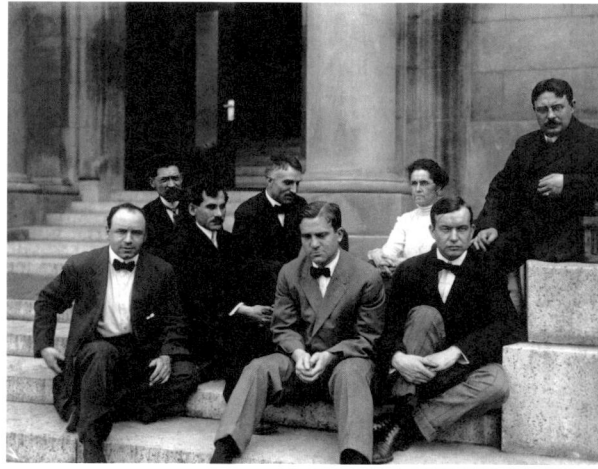

Chemist P.A.T. Levene (third from left) and members of his laboratory.

Three scientists working in P.A.T. Levene's Founder's Hall chemistry laboratory (from left to right): Walter Jacobs, Donald Van Slyke, and Gustave Meyer. (1908)

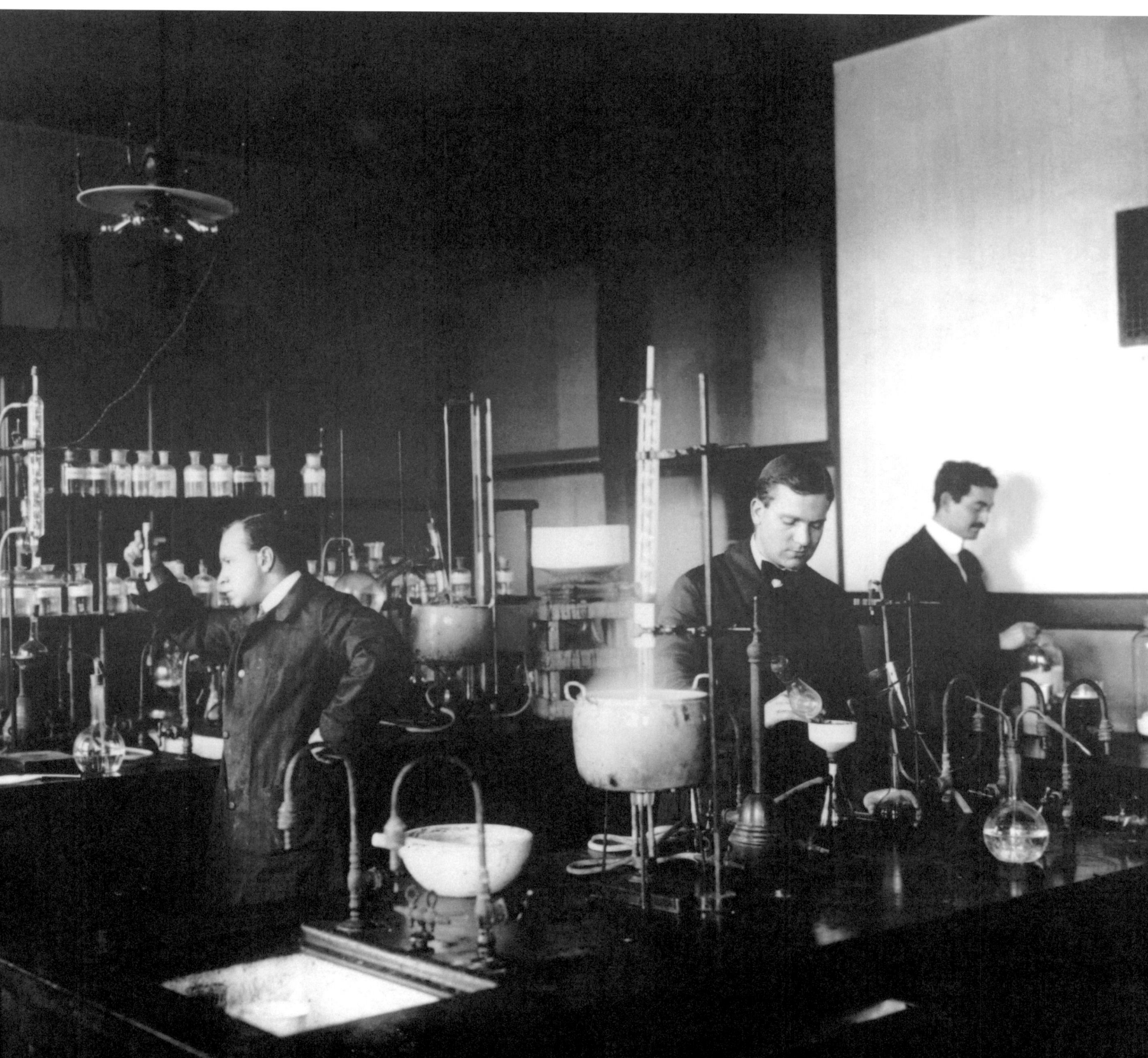

Flexner's firm belief in allowing his senior investigators to follow their own research instincts made the Institute different from its European predecessors such as the Koch and Pasteur Institutes, where all scientists carried out the research plan of the great man at the head of the institution. Flexner's conviction was based on the advice of many scientific leaders, and he paid particular attention to that of Anton Dohrn, founder of the Naples Zoological Station. Dohrn explained to Flexner: "Men work here in a dozen different branches of biological science; can I be an authority on them all? No, no, give them perfect freedom; let them search where and how they will; help them in every way you can, but do not pretend to be master over them."

Simon Flexner and John D. Rockefeller Jr. worked closely together in the early years of the Institute, and through this association Flexner converted Rockefeller Jr. to the view that scientists had to be left alone in order to accomplish their work. In part this reflected the fact that the Institute's credibility rested on there being no interference—or even the appearance of it—from the Rockefellers. But Rockefeller Jr. also was convinced of Flexner's larger point about the nature of science as a scholarly endeavor, and he played an active role in ensuring the independence of the Institute's researchers. In 1910 the separation of business management from scientific oversight became institutionalized when the original Board of Directors split into a Board of Trustees, chaired by Frederick Gates, and a Board of Scientific Directors, led by William Welch.

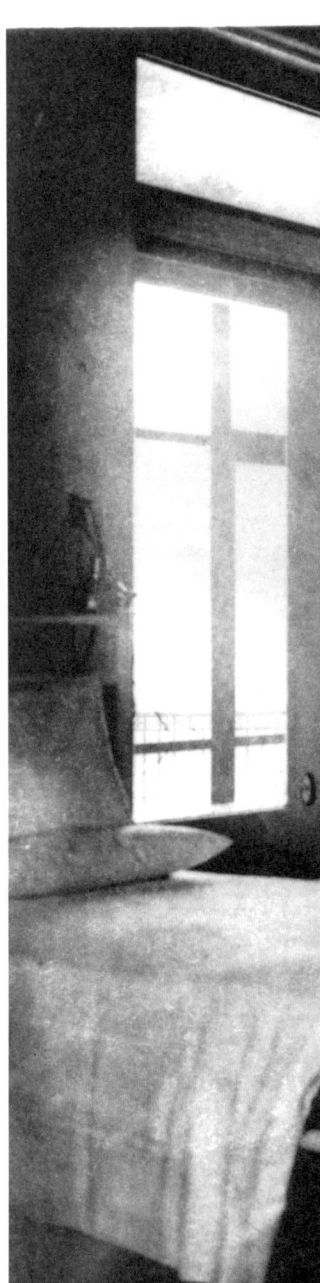

The Hospital

With research laboratories in place, Flexner proceeded with the next element in his plan for the Institute—a research hospital. The Hospital was part of his earliest proposal. He wrote, "In order that [the problems of human disease] be not neglected, there should be attached to the Institute a hospital for the study of special groups of cases of disease. This hospital should be modern and fully equipped, but it need not be large. It should attempt to provide only for selected cases of disease."

Flexner's early plan for a research hospital was influenced by the ideas of Board member Christian Herter. The two of them envisioned the Hospital as a testing ground for ideas developed in the laboratories, and as a source of specimens such as blood and urine from patients with specific diseases. In 1907 Rockefeller promised $500,000 for Hospital construction. Herter would have become the first head of

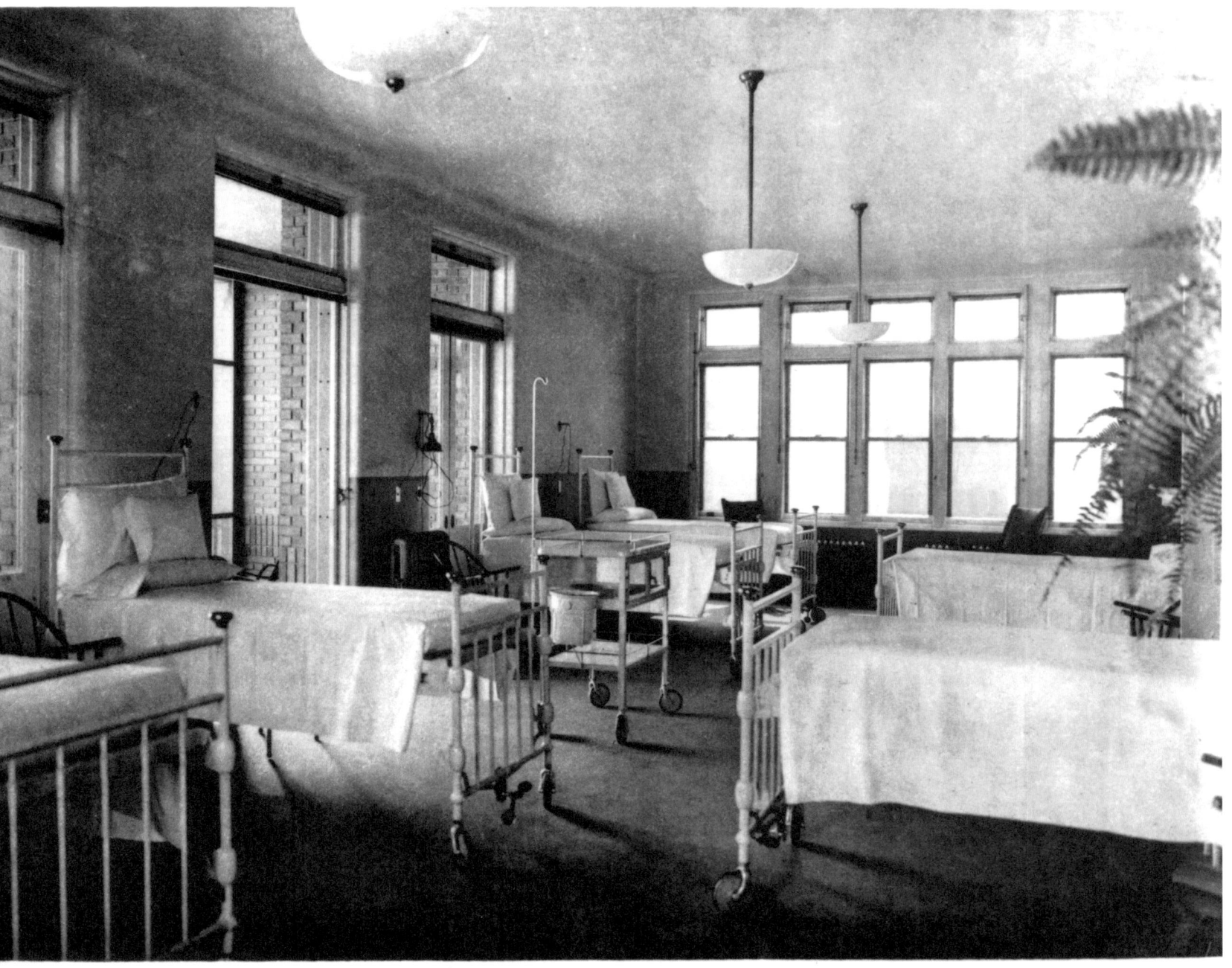

Wards in The Rockefeller Institute's hospital, where only patients with diseases under study were admitted, were smaller than at other hospitals. (1911)

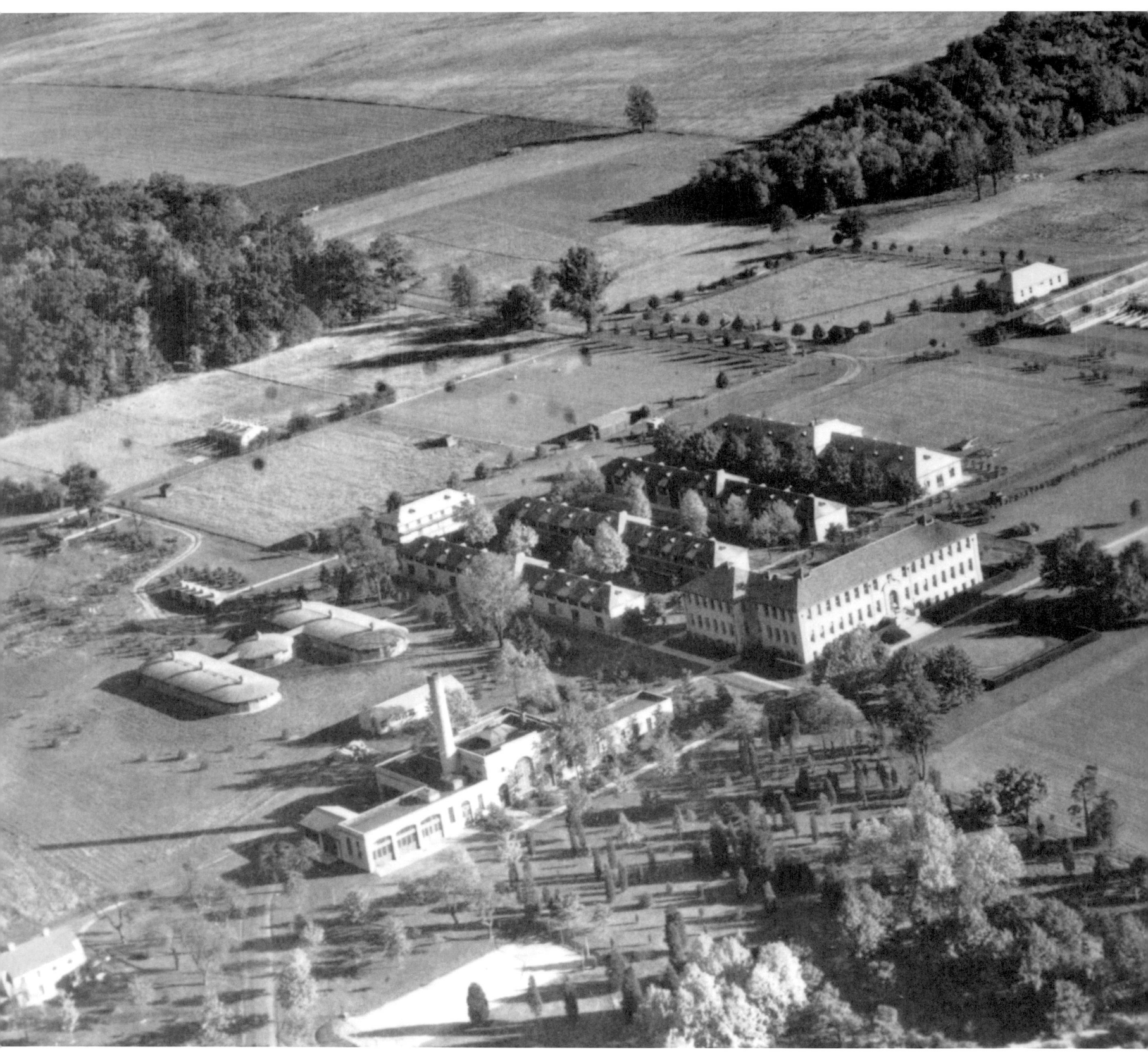

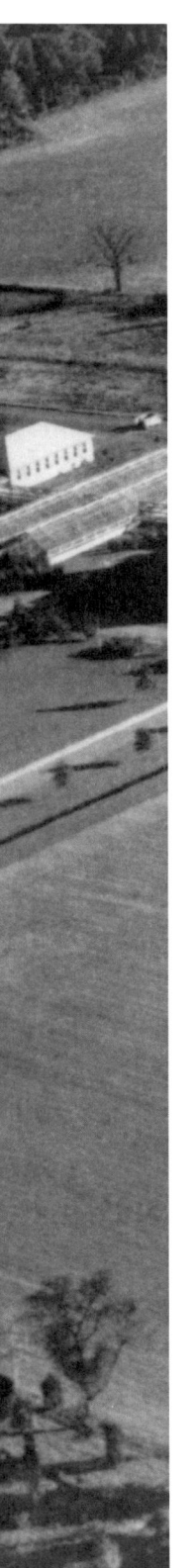

The Rockefeller Institute's department of animal pathology, later animal and plant pathology, was located in Princeton, New Jersey, east of Carnegie Lake and adjacent to Princeton University.

the Hospital but for his own tragic illness—he suffered from myasthenia gravis, an autoimmune disorder. The Board had to look for someone else to fill the job.

In 1908 Rufus Cole became the first head of the Hospital. Like Flexner, he had received his medical education at Johns Hopkins. Cole adopted a new approach to the running of a hospital, different from that first planned. Flexner and Herter had separated laboratory science and patient care, emulating the organization of the few hospitals in the country where research was conducted. In their scheme, research was aimed mainly at improving the diagnosis of disease. Cole combined these functions and focused on understanding the underlying causes of disease. In the Rockefeller Hospital, physician-scientists would both care for patients and study them, having their own laboratories alongside the wards. Observations of patients would suggest research questions that could be answered in the lab, and Hospital physicians would carry out their own independent research. Freed from the teaching responsibilities of a medical school and barred from outside practice, these physicians would devote all their time to clinical research. Furthermore, they would focus on particular diseases. In the early years of the Hospital these included poliomyelitis, lobar pneumonia, syphilis, and heart disease.

The Hospital opened in October 1910 as a department of the Institute separate from the laboratories. At this time John D. Rockefeller made a donation that brought the Institute's endowment to more than $6 million. The Hospital's physicians had the status of full members of the Institute, like other laboratory heads. From its inception, The Rockefeller Institute's Hospital was foremost among the few places in the United States where clinical research was practiced; it was the only institution devoted exclusively to it and was paramount in spreading this ideal. By the 1950s more than 100 physician-scientists who had worked at the Rockefeller Hospital had gone on to become professors in medical schools in the United States and abroad.

The focus of the Institute as a whole remained the study of infectious disease, and until 1913 it was limited to human diseases. In that year, however, an infectious animal disease—hog cholera—was costing farmers in the western United States tens of millions of dollars. The Institute received an offer of $25,000 to investigate this disease. But rather than set research priorities on a disease-by-disease basis, the Board of Scientific Directors supported the establishment of an extension of the Institute, a department of animal pathology in Princeton, New Jersey.

With the support of a $1 million pledge from John D. Rockefeller and a $1 million appropriation from the Rockefeller Foundation, the facility was built in 1916. Theobald Smith, earlier reluctant to take on the directorship of the entire Institute, now relinquished his Harvard professorship to direct the department of animal pathology. The Princeton facility became the site of groundbreaking research in virology, and the Nobel Prize–winning chemists John H. Northrop and Wendell M. Stanley carried out their work on the purification and crystallization of enzymes and viruses there. When the department of animal pathology was closed in 1949, many of the senior investigators joined the Institute staff in New York.

At its founding and in its first decades, The Rockefeller Institute for Medical Research advanced a unique approach to tackling the scientific problems of infectious diseases and was far more influential than its modest campus and small faculty might suggest. The Kaiser Wilhelm Institute, founded in Germany in 1911, was patterned directly after The Rockefeller Institute, and research centers in the United States also looked to Rockefeller as a model; the Memorial Institute for Infectious Diseases in Chicago and the Phipps Institute for the Study, Treatment, and Prevention of Tuberculosis in Philadelphia are two examples. Other new organizations, such as the Medical Research Council in England, sought Flexner's advice.

Reflecting on the first 25 years of the Institute's history, Simon Flexner could already say that "profound changes have taken place within the United States in medical research and in the hospital care and study of the sick. There is appreciation of the fact that the contributions of The Rockefeller Institute to these constructive changes have been significant."

FOUNDING

A Closer Look: The Rockefeller Institute for Medical Research

The Institute Goes to War 28

A New Kind of Hero 31

Making New York's Milk Supply Safe 32

Rockefeller's World-Famous Microbe Hunters 34

Howard Hughes, the Institute, and the University 36

The Philanthropy of John D. Rockefeller 38

A Hub for Scientific Exchange 41

Building a Campus 42

John D. Rockefeller Visits the Institute 45

Hidden Histories 46

Simon Flexner 49

The Institute Goes to War

After the United States entered World War I in April 1917, work at the Institute was given over to the war effort. A War Demonstration Hospital was built on the campus with funds from the Rockefeller Foundation. The 16 wooden buildings were designed to be portable, for quick assembly at the front. At the Institute they became classrooms for training military medical officers.

Here the Nobel Prize–winning surgeon Alexis Carrel, assisted by French and American military surgeons, gave instruction in a novel method for cleansing and suturing wounds. Carrel had developed the method earlier in the war while he was in France. It called for radical surgical removal of injured tissues and the flushing of wounds with an antiseptic solution developed by British biochemist Henry Dakin, which was essentially dilute chlorine bleach. Between August 1917 and March 1919 a new group of medical officers arrived at the Institute every two weeks for the course.

Teaching courses in bacteriology, clinical chemistry, and the techniques of pathology became an important task of the Institute. In August 1918 the War Department commissioned the Institute as an Army post, and nearly all qualified staff went into uniform. Simon Flexner continued his directorship with the rank of Lieutenant Colonel.

Research also continued, directed toward the problems of war. Peyton Rous and his associates found a practical method of preserving whole blood for use in transfusion—in essence, making possible the first blood bank. Other work was aimed at producing serums against meningitis and dysentery, and seeking a treatment for gas gangrene.

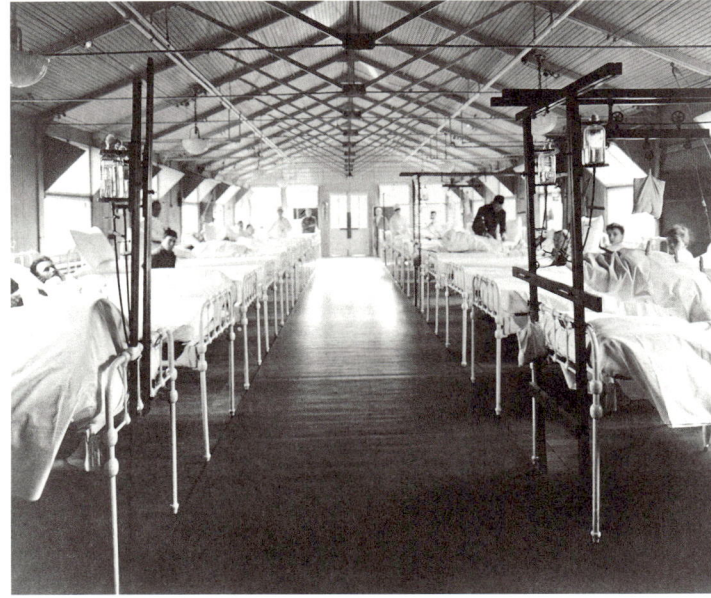

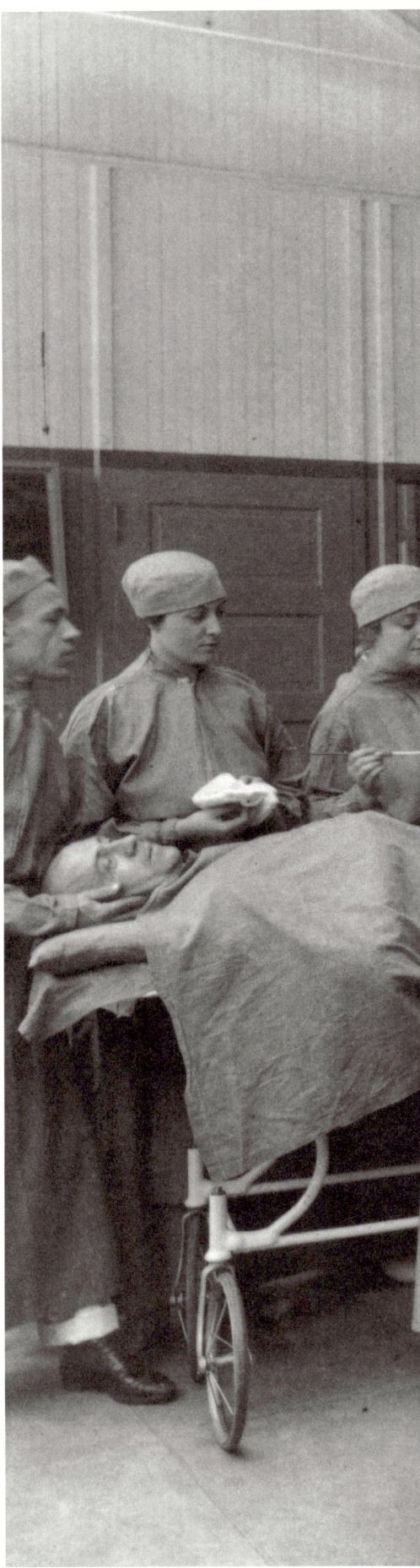

Alexis Carrel (standing at center, with white cap) trained military doctors in surgical techniques during World War I (right). A ward in one of the War Demonstration Hospital buildings (left).

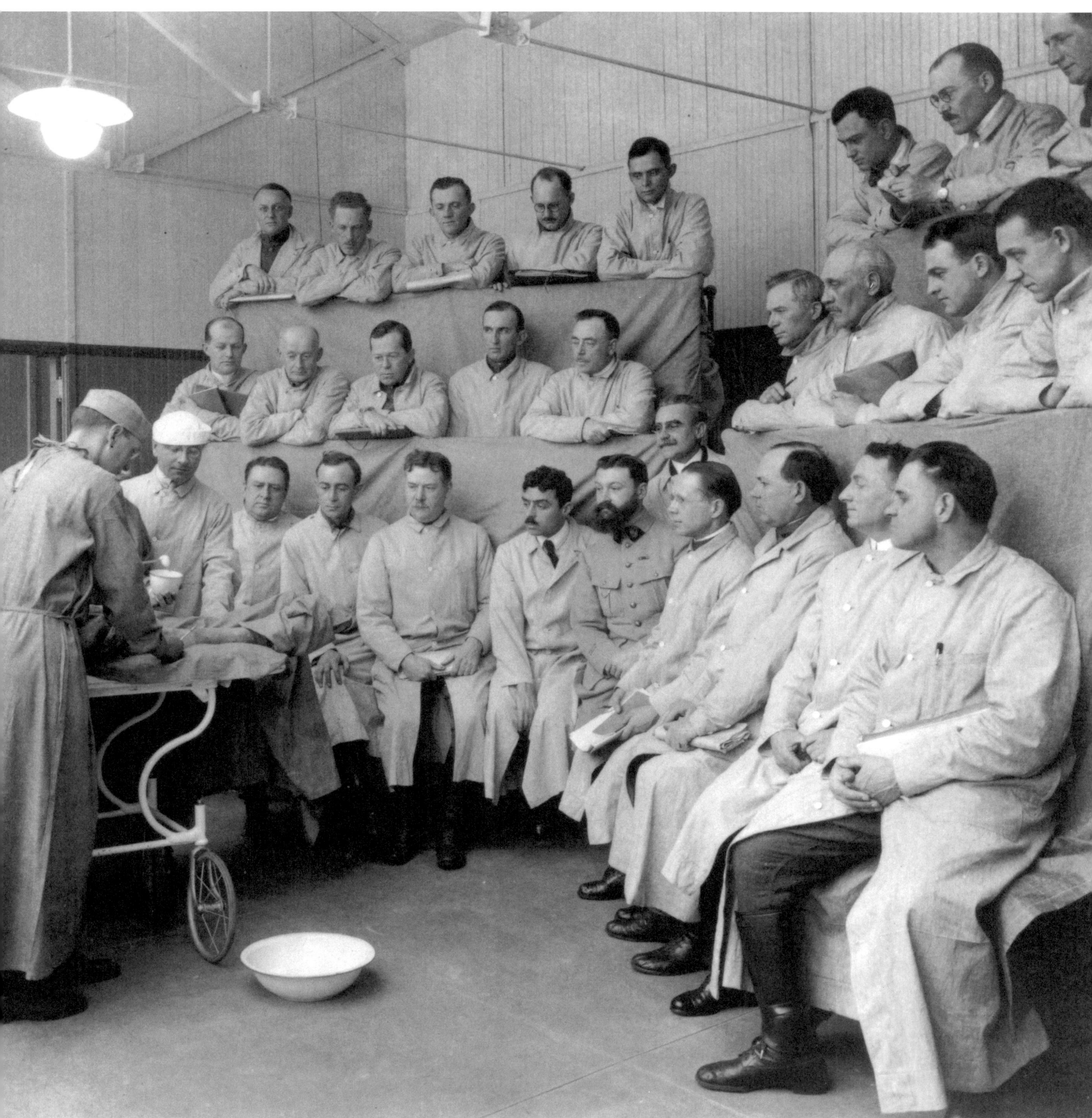

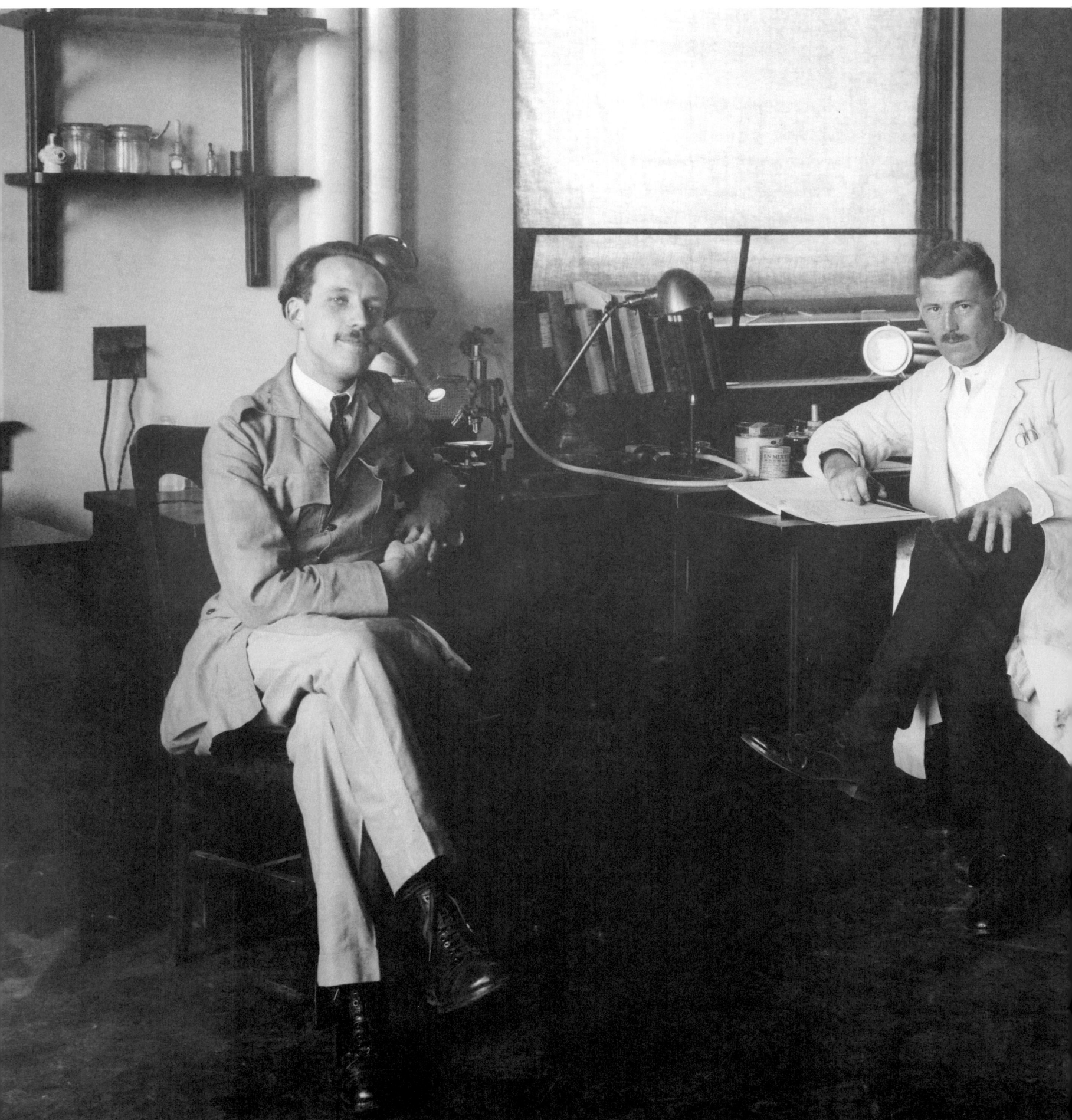

A New Kind of Hero

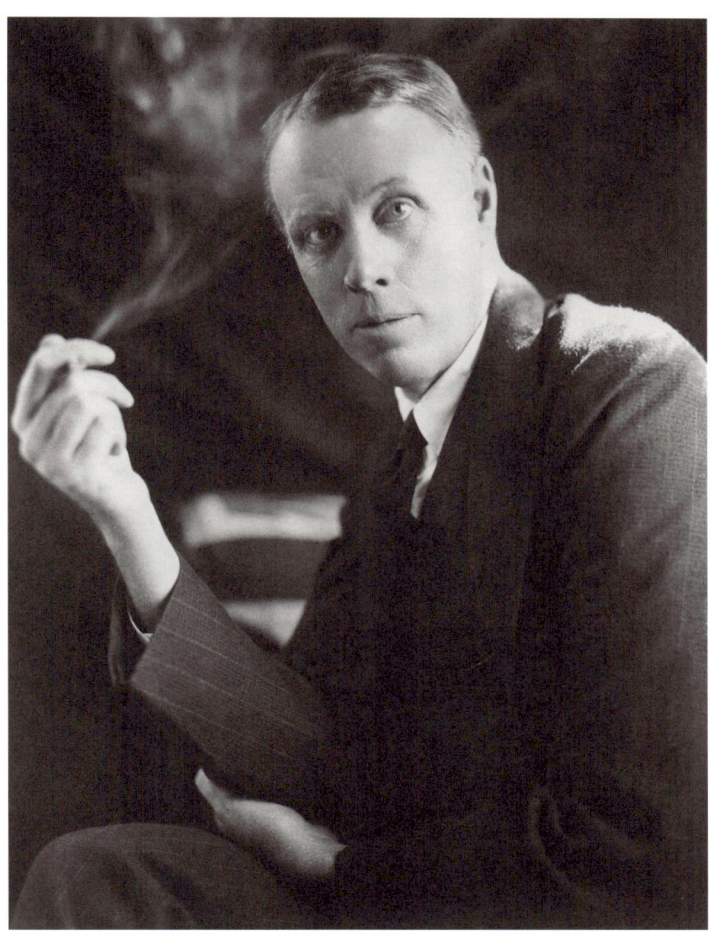

In 1930 Sinclair Lewis became the first American to receive the Nobel Prize for literature. Far left: Paul de Kruif (seated at right) and Belgian bacteriologist Leon E. Gratia worked in Simon Flexner's laboratory. (1921)

Sinclair Lewis's novel *Arrowsmith*, published in 1925, introduced a new kind of hero to the American public—the research scientist. The story revolves around Martin Arrowsmith's moral struggle between the material rewards of practicing medicine, portrayed as dishonest in light of medicine's limited ability to cure disease early in the century, and the integrity and idealism of basic scientific research. *Arrowsmith* won a 1926 Pulitzer Prize, which Lewis refused on the grounds that "all prizes, like all titles, are dangerous." The novel was made into a film in 1932.

Lewis wrote the book with the close consultation of Paul de Kruif, who had worked in Simon Flexner's laboratory at The Rockefeller Institute for two years beginning in 1920. De Kruif gave up research for popular science writing—in fact, Flexner fired him for publishing an anonymous critique of medical science in a widely circulated magazine. He went on to write *The Microbe Hunters*, a collection of tales that chronicle the development of bacteriology from Leeuwenhoek—the first to see single-celled organisms with a microscope in the late 1600s—through the scientists of the early 20th century.

For *Arrowsmith*, de Kruif provided Lewis with character sketches based on scientists he knew. Martin Arrowsmith's mentor Max Gottlieb was a composite of Rockefeller's Jacques Loeb and F.G. Novy, de Kruif's doctoral advisor at the University of Michigan. Loeb's philosophy, and his habit of lecturing to his colleagues, is evident in Gottlieb's paeans to physical chemistry. Gottlieb tells Arrowsmith: "Physical chemistry is power, it is exactness, it is life." The character Terry Wickett shared attributes with Rockefeller's John Northrop. And The Rockefeller Institute itself and its director Simon Flexner were fictionalized as the novel's McGurk Institute and the character A. DeWitt Tubbs.

Making New York's Milk Supply Safe

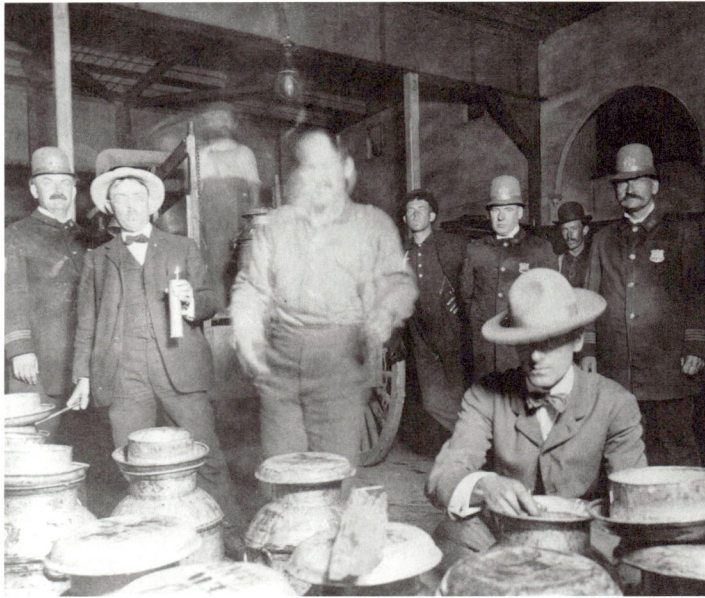

At the turn of the 20th century epidemics of diarrhea among infants and toddlers swept into New York City each year with the warm summer weather. Contaminated, unrefrigerated milk was thought to be the source of the problem. Among the first research grants awarded by The Rockefeller Institute, in 1901 and 1902, was a study of the bacterial content of milk in collaboration with the New York City Department of Health.

The study compared the numbers of bacteria in pasteurized and unpasteurized milk, and correlated the results with the health of babies who drank the milk. Milk samples were taken, dairies inspected, and infant health monitored in homes and in children's hospitals. Bacterial counts from milk sold from open cans to tenement dwellers proved shockingly high, and researchers even found "Germs Swarming in City's Purest Milk" according to newspaper headlines. The research prompted the health department to reform the handling and sale of milk even before the study was finished.

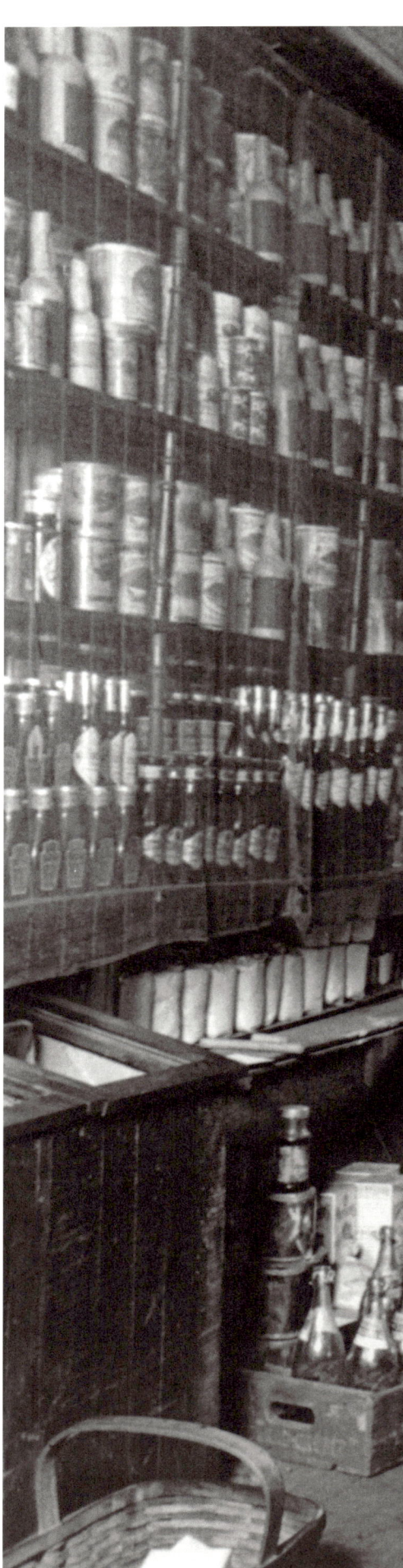

Inspectors from the New York City Department of Health took samples of milk as it was delivered by dairymen to the city and inside grocery stores.

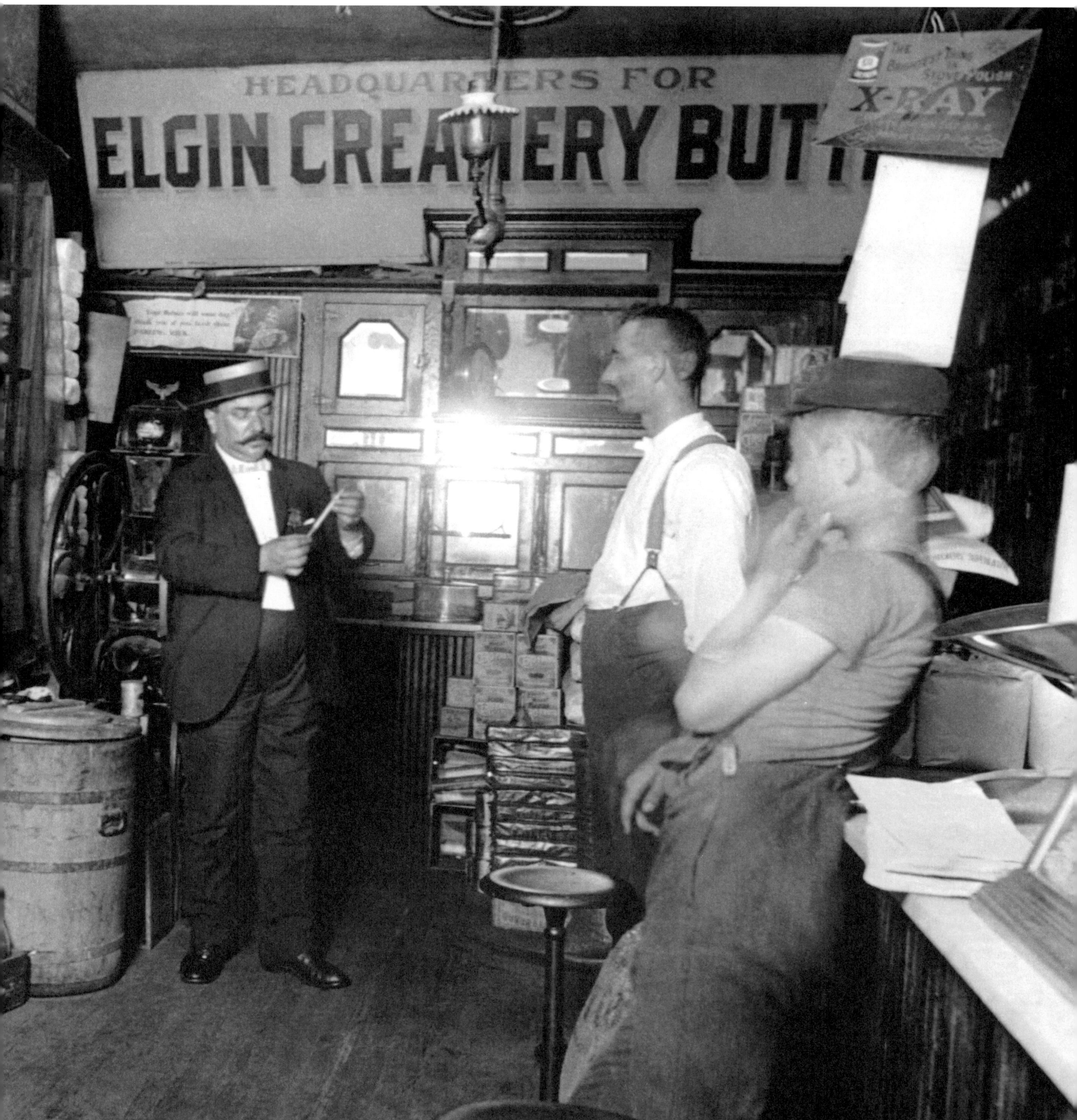

Rockefeller's World-Famous Microbe Hunters

The Rockefeller Institute for Medical Research gained national recognition early in its history. Rockefeller's name alone made establishment of the Institute big news. But soon the Institute's scientists and their work made headlines on their own. Although chemists and other researchers pursued groundbreaking work, those doing microbial detective work—hunting down and isolating disease-causing organisms—captured the public imagination.

The Institute's director, Simon Flexner, was the first. In 1905 the New York City Board of Health asked Flexner to investigate an epidemic of cerebrospinal meningitis. To treat the disease Flexner developed a serum that was injected directly into the spinal cord.

During a 1907 epidemic in Ohio the serum was credited with reducing the rate of meningitis deaths from three in four cases to one in four. The New York *World* announced, "Cure is Found for Meningitis with John D.'s Aid." The serum's success helped convince Rockefeller to support the construction of the Hospital at the Institute. The serum itself remained the only means for reducing deaths from this disease for decades until the advent of sulfa drugs and antibiotics.

Flexner's protégé Hideyo Noguchi achieved both fame and notoriety. Noguchi, the son of impoverished Japanese peasants, had attained some medical education by the time he met Simon Flexner in 1899. Noguchi interpreted Flexner's words of encouragement as an invitation to the United States, and when Noguchi appeared on the doorstep of Flexner's laboratory at the University of Pennsylvania, Flexner took him in.

Noguchi followed Flexner to Rockefeller, setting to work on what seemed a brilliant career in microbiology, culturing for the first time organisms such as syphilis and other spirochetes, the polio and rabies viruses, vaccinia virus, and the infectious agent of Oroya fever, a disease that had killed thousands during outbreaks in mountainous regions of South America. Some of his work proved durable; other results were later discredited. At the time, however, scientific leaders around the world applauded Noguchi's achievements, inviting him to deliver lectures and honoring him at banquets.

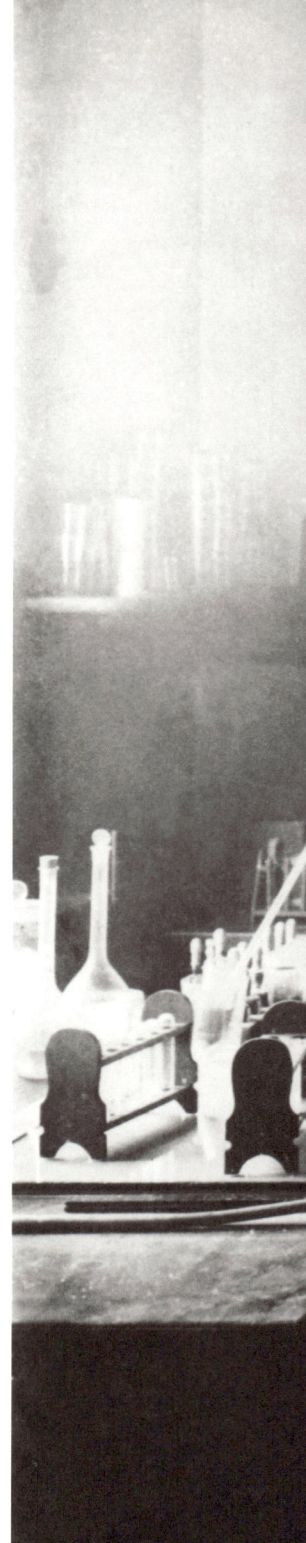

Hideyo Noguchi gained both fame and notoriety in his globe-trotting pursuit of disease-causing microbes.

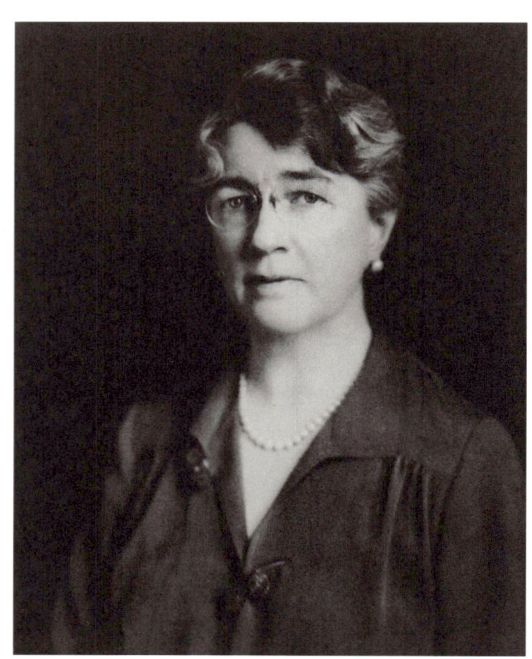

Louise Pearce developed a drug to treat African sleeping sickness. She received an M.D. from the Johns Hopkins Medical School before coming to work in Simon Flexner's laboratory at The Rockefeller Institute.

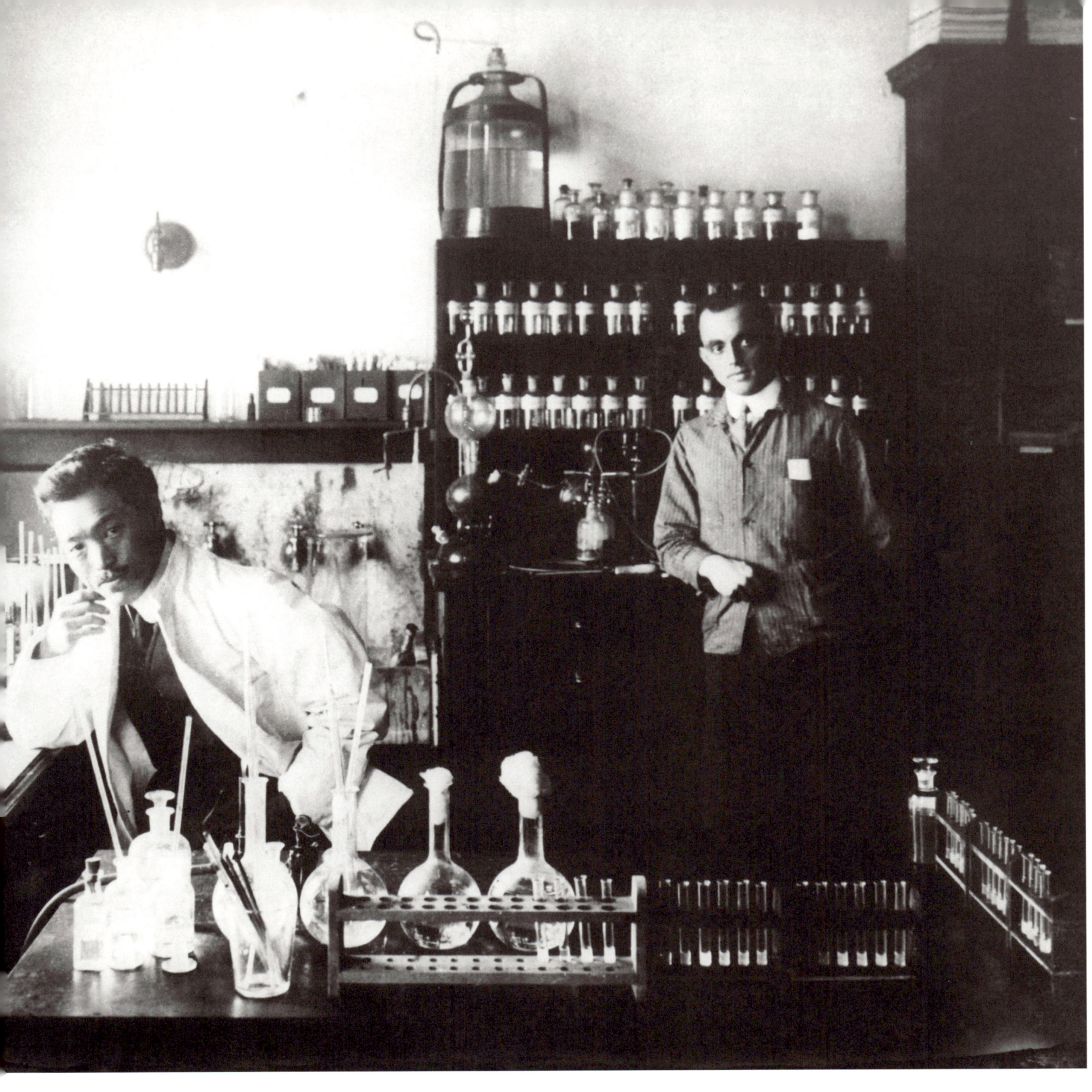

Noguchi's grandest pursuit—the search for the organism that causes yellow fever—brought about both his scientific downfall and tragic death. Noguchi believed the infectious agent to be a spirochete he had isolated from yellow fever patients in Ecuador, but others doubted his results. In 1927 Noguchi boarded a ship to West Africa to search for the organism there. Within a few months, after having discovered his earlier results to be wrong, he became infected with yellow fever and died.

At about the same time that Noguchi began his work on yellow fever, other members of Flexner's laboratory set about synthesizing a drug to treat African sleeping sickness, or trypanosomiasis, which is caused by a blood parasite. By refining an arsenic-containing compound used to treat syphilis, they came up with a drug called Tryparsamide. Louise Pearce traveled to the then Belgian Congo in 1920 to test its effectiveness in human cases of sleeping sickness. The treatment was so successful that Pearce and her colleagues were decorated by the Belgian government.

Howard Hughes, the Institute, and the University

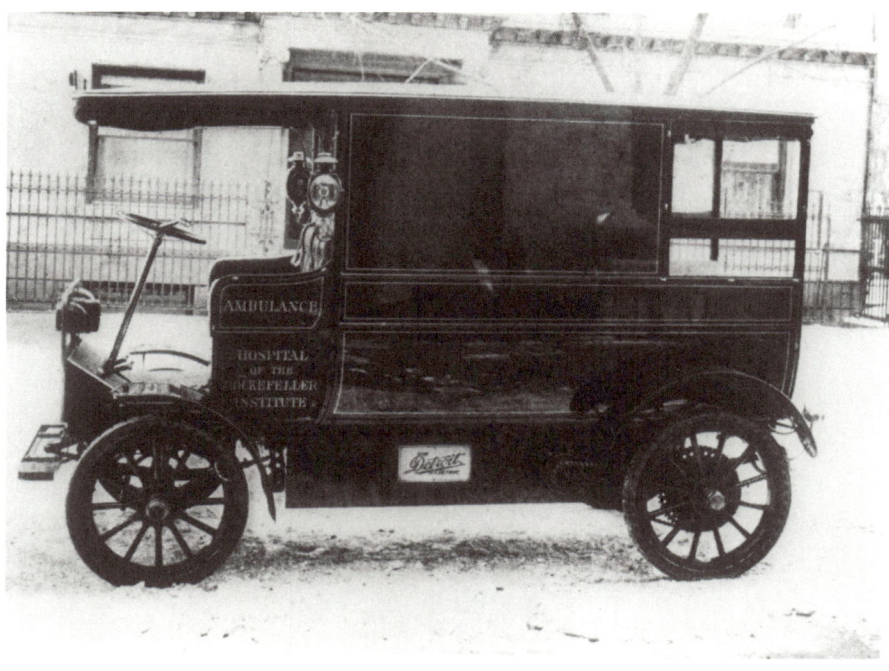

Entrepreneur, aviator, and movie mogul Howard Hughes had a longstanding interest in medical research, culminating in the founding of the Howard Hughes Medical Institute in 1953. Today, a dozen Rockefeller University professors are also HHMI investigators. But the relationship between the University and Hughes—both the man and the Institute—goes back more than eight decades. Purnell Choppin, a former HHMI president and former Rockefeller faculty member, tells the story this way:

"There was a wonderful switchboard operator for over 50 years at RU, Frank Capellino. Sometime around 1915, Capellino encountered a distraught looking gentleman in the lobby of Founder's Hall. He asked the man if he could help him. The man said he had come from Texas because his nephew was quite ill with some kind of meningitis. RU had already become well-known for its infectious disease research. Frank sent the man to the young clinician Dr. Henry Chickering. At that time in his career, Chickering was not particularly interested in interrupting his work to go to Texas, which is what this gentleman wanted him to do.

"The visitor returned to Capellino to say good-bye and relate Chickering's rejection. Capellino then called Simon Flexner to ask him if he would talk to Chickering on the visitor's behalf. Flexner persuaded Chickering to go to the sick boy, Howard Hughes. The boy's uncle, Rupert Hughes, was very grateful.

"Decades later, David Rockefeller wrote to Mr. Hughes, who by that time was a total recluse. Rockefeller suggested that Hughes' survival was likely due to Chickering's help. Hughes never responded to the letter. I like to say that, ultimately, there was an answer to that letter."

That answer came in the late 1980s in the form of an agreement between Rockefeller and the Howard Hughes Medical Institute that initiated construction of a new laboratory building on campus and the hiring of joint Rockefeller–HHMI faculty.

An ambulance of the Hospital of The Rockefeller Institute (left), and the Hospital entrance as it looked in 1911. Pneumonia, syphilis, and polio were among the first diseases studied at the Hospital.

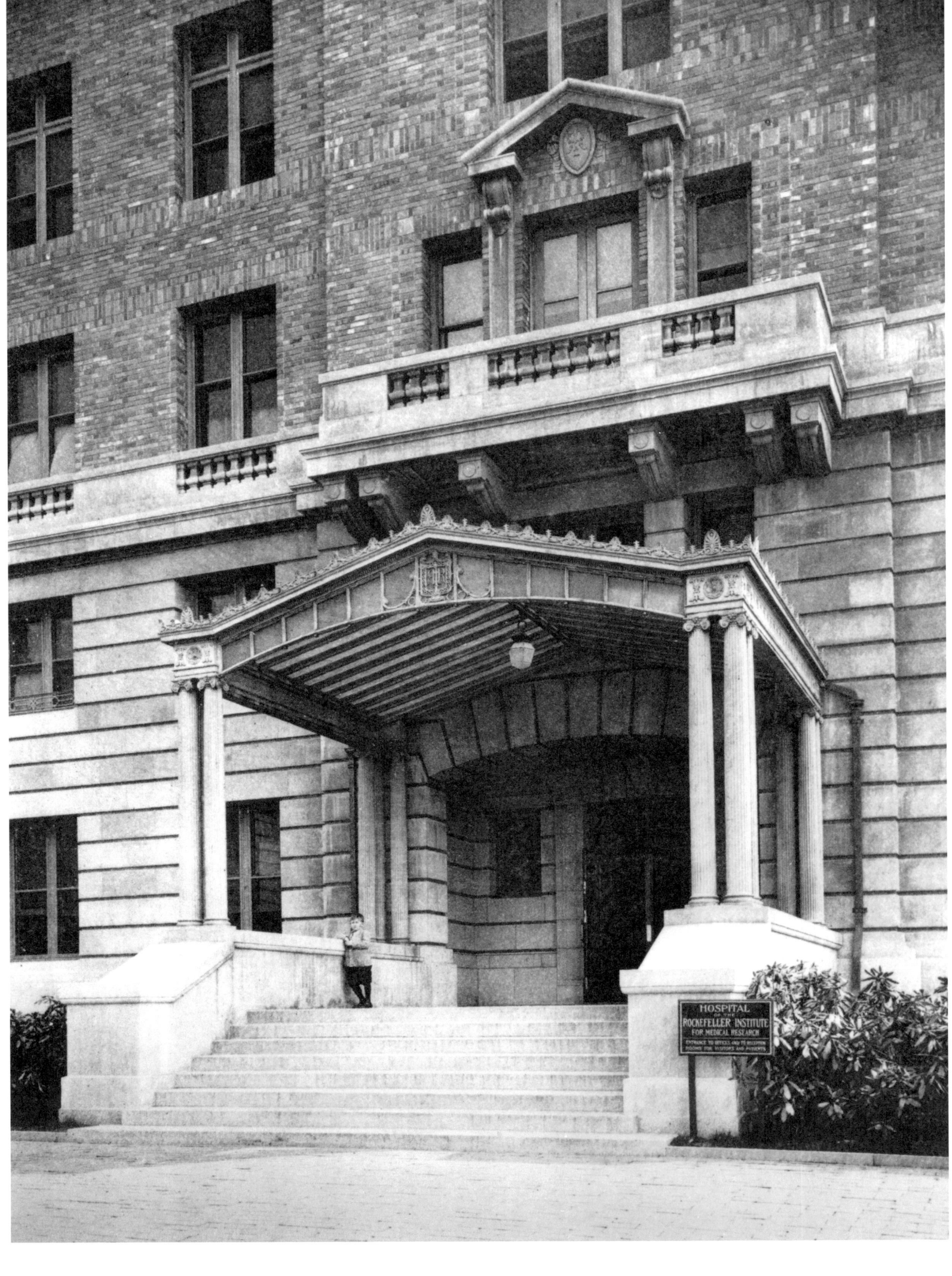

The Philanthropy of John D. Rockefeller

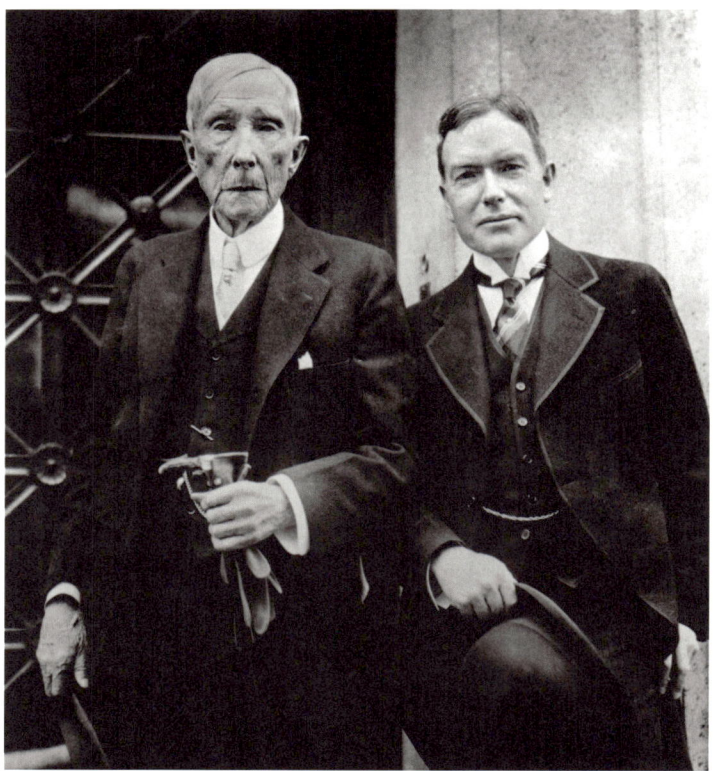

John D. Rockefeller amassed the largest fortune in history with the profits of his Standard Oil Company. At the peak of his wealth in 1913, he was worth nearly a billion dollars. Rockefeller also was a devout Baptist and, in keeping with his religious upbringing, he believed that wealth conferred the responsibility to give. The systematic way in which Rockefeller dispersed his fortune—his business of benevolence—was at the vanguard of a new kind of philanthropy at the turn of the 20th century.

In fact, Rockefeller had donated to charity from the first paycheck he received working as a bookkeeper while he was still a teenager. As he gained wealth and fame, he was besieged by requests for money—as many as a half million letters a year. To deal with this volume of requests and to accomplish what he believed to be the greatest benefit with his philanthropy Rockefeller applied his prodigious managerial skills.

In the 19th century philanthropy had been a matter of small gifts to individuals. The vast fortunes accumulated at the end of the century by magnates in oil, steel, banking, and railroads spurred a new kind of philanthropy. Gifts were made on a grander scale, reaching beyond the benefactors' local communities and transcending sectarianism. Rockefeller based his gifts on a system of rational analysis. He evaluated projects on their potential to succeed and benefit society in the long term. Rockefeller also focused on building institutions that would take on a life of their own once established. He did not want to foster dependency on his future donations.

This strategy took shape with Rockefeller's donations to help found Spelman Seminary, later renamed Spelman College. In 1882 Spelman was a small school for emancipated female slaves set up in an Atlanta church basement. Rockefeller donated funds for its campus site and other facilities, but he made sure that the school would look beyond his help for support. Rockefeller applied the same principle to his donations for founding the University of Chicago in the 1890s. In addition, he would not allow the school to name any building after him, or even to use a lamp on its seal, for fear that doing so would be taken as an advertisement for Standard Oil.

John D. Rockefeller stayed away from the day-to-day affairs of the Institute, leaving his son John D. Rockefeller Jr., who became chairman of the Board of Trustees, to keep him informed.

In this book, known as Ledger A, John D. Rockefeller recorded his earliest charitable donations.

Spelman and the University of Chicago were both Baptist organizations. With his third foray into institution building—The Rockefeller Institute for Medical Research—Rockefeller reached beyond his church affiliation and ventured into new philanthropic territory. The patronage of science through private philanthropy was a new idea, as unconventional as the notion that systematic medical research could lead to cures for disease. Rockefeller's commitment to the Institute may also have been strengthened by a rival; in 1902 Andrew Carnegie incorporated the Carnegie Institute of Washington. While not exclusively focused on medical discoveries, the Carnegie Institute's chartered purpose was research for the improvement of mankind.

In the years after The Rockefeller Institute was established, Rockefeller's support of science grew. In 1909 he founded the Rockefeller Sanitary Commission, with the mission of eradicating hookworm disease in the southern United States. The Rockefeller Foundation and International Health Board, both established in 1913, extended this work globally. Public health and disease control programs became a mainstay of the Foundation's work, leading in 1935 to the development of a vaccine against yellow fever, which was developed in Rockefeller Foundation laboratories on the campus of the Institute. In the 1930s and 1940s the Foundation turned to funding basic research in what would come to be called molecular biology. Spending nearly $100 million in that period, the Foundation was the largest underwriter of the life sciences before the Second World War. By the time John D. Rockefeller died in 1937 at the age of 97, he had given $540 million to the causes of health, education, and public welfare.

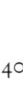

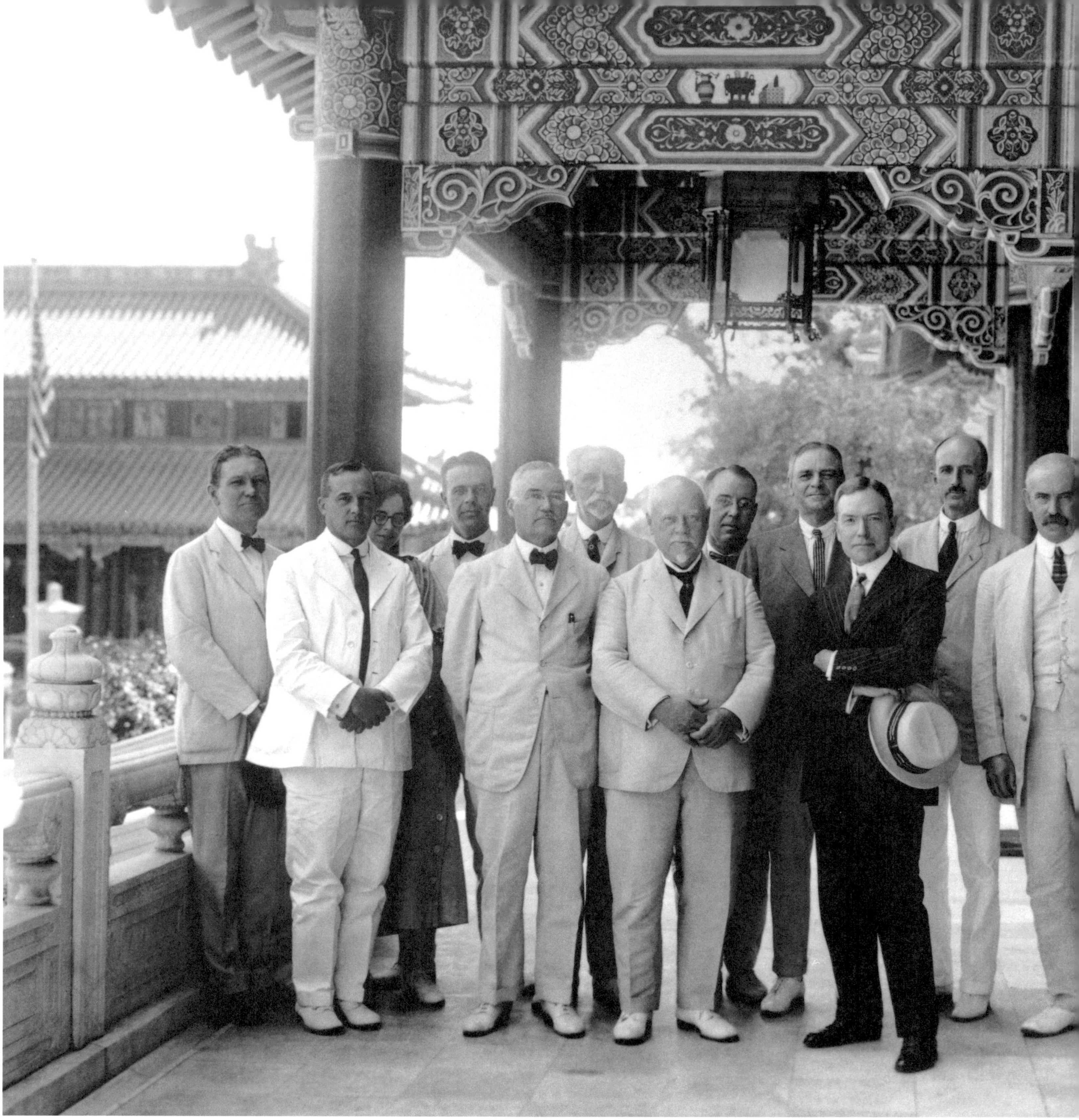

A Hub for Scientific Exchange

At the beginning of the 20th century the established centers for scientific research remained in Europe, and young scientists traveled there for training in the latest techniques and knowledge. Part of the Institute's avowed mission, indeed, was to rescue the United States from the backwaters of medical science. With its New York City location and its well-connected staff, the Institute quickly became a crossroads for scientific exchange.

Simon Flexner's position of high regard in national and international scientific circles helped make the Institute a magnet for outstanding researchers. When he became director of the Institute Flexner recruited an international scientific staff. Meltzer and Levene were both born in Russia, Carrel was French, and Loeb came from Germany. Flexner himself spent much of 1903 and 1904 on a tour of European research laboratories, learning about their work and organization, and educating himself in the latest advances in biochemistry.

Flexner nurtured a pool of talent from which the Institute could draw. As a charter member of the Board of Directors of the Rockefeller Foundation, he oversaw fellowships awarded to young scientists through the National Research Council. Through this work he monitored the progress of upcoming generations of researchers.

The Rockefeller Foundation forged another international link for the Institute when it created the Peking Union Medical College in 1915, in an effort to introduce Western medicine to China. Flexner belonged to the Foundation's China Medical Board, and the Medical College's first director, Franklin C. McLean, was recruited from the Rockefeller Hospital. Scientific exchange continued in the 1920s and 1930s, as members of the Institute went to China as visiting professors and graduates of the College came to the Institute for further study.

Researchers seeking postgraduate training arrived from around the United States and from Europe and China. In the first half of the century, before formal postdoctoral training became routine, a stint at the Institute became almost a prerequisite—although an unofficial one—for young scientists pursuing a research career. The concentration of renowned researchers, and opportunities for short-term research appointments, drew a steady stream of fresh ideas and scientific expertise to the Institute. The laboratory of Peter Olitsky included scientists from so many countries in the 1920s that Institute staff referred to it as "the League of Nations."

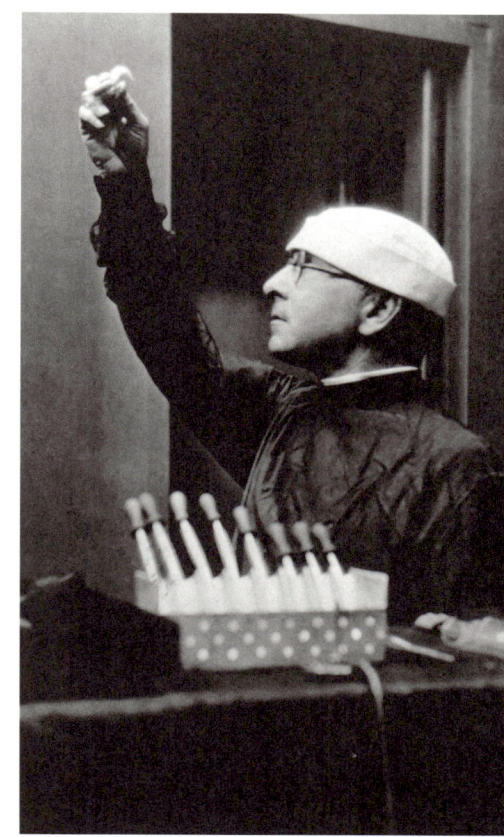

War also opened up opportunities for international scientific collaborations. During World War I, when the Institute became, in effect, an Army facility, the ties forged between the Institute and Army personnel who trained there spread Rockefeller's reputation and continued far into the future. Rockefeller professor emeritus and Nobel laureate R. Bruce Merrifield recalls that his doctoral advisor, M.S. Dunn, had taken the clinical chemistry course with Donald Van Slyke at the Institute's War Demonstration Hospital. In the late 1940s, when Rockefeller chemist D. Wayne Woolley had an opening for a researcher in his laboratory, he contacted Dunn, who recommended Merrifield.

Representatives of the Rockefeller Foundation visited the Peking Union Medical College. At center, with the goatee, is William H. Welch. Next to him, in the dark suit, is John D. Rockefeller Jr.

Frenchman Alexis Carrel headed a laboratory at the Institute from 1906 to 1941.

Building a Campus

To design the first laboratory of The Rockefeller Institute, the Board of Directors hired the Boston firm of Shepley, Rutan, and Coolidge. The architect Charles Coolidge, in particular, had already achieved recognition for his buildings on college campuses, among them the University of Chicago and the Harvard Medical School. Now called Founder's Hall, the first building on Rockefeller's campus was completed in 1906. In 1974 it was designated a National Historic Landmark and added to the National Register of Historic Places.

A different firm—York and Sawyer—built the Rockefeller Hospital and the original Isolation Ward (1910), later to become the Nurses Residence. But the Institute's administration turned again to Coolidge for Flexner Hall (1917), Welch Hall (1929), and Theobald Smith Hall (1930).

Early campus planning also called for a boiler house—now called the power house—so that the Institute would be self-sufficient for power. Coal for the boilers was delivered from barges on the East River. In 1915 workers spent months dynamiting the site's natural stone ledge and constructing a new wall that encloses the power house and marks the edge of campus. This wall, which today lines the Franklin D. Roosevelt Drive, is built of Manhattan schist taken from the site.

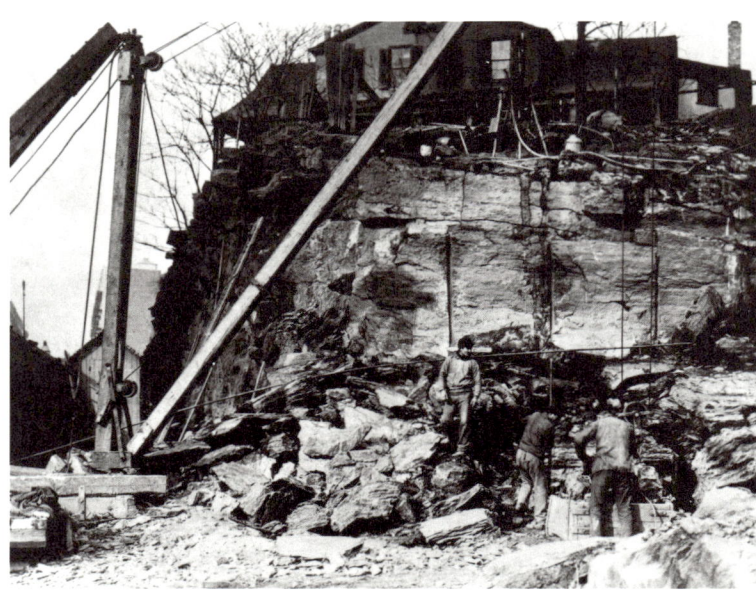

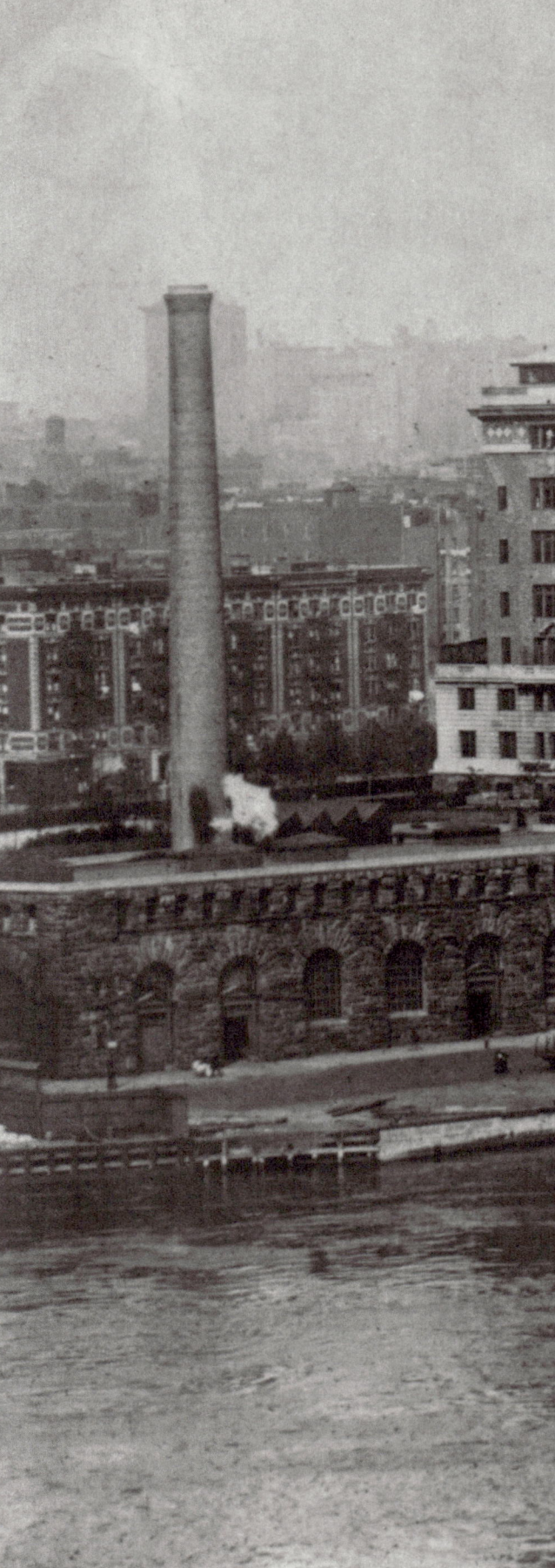

Workers remove stone from the Institute's site (left). (c. 1903) The power house, the Hospital, Nurse's Residence, Founder's Hall, and Flexner Hall are visible in this 1920 view from the East River (right).

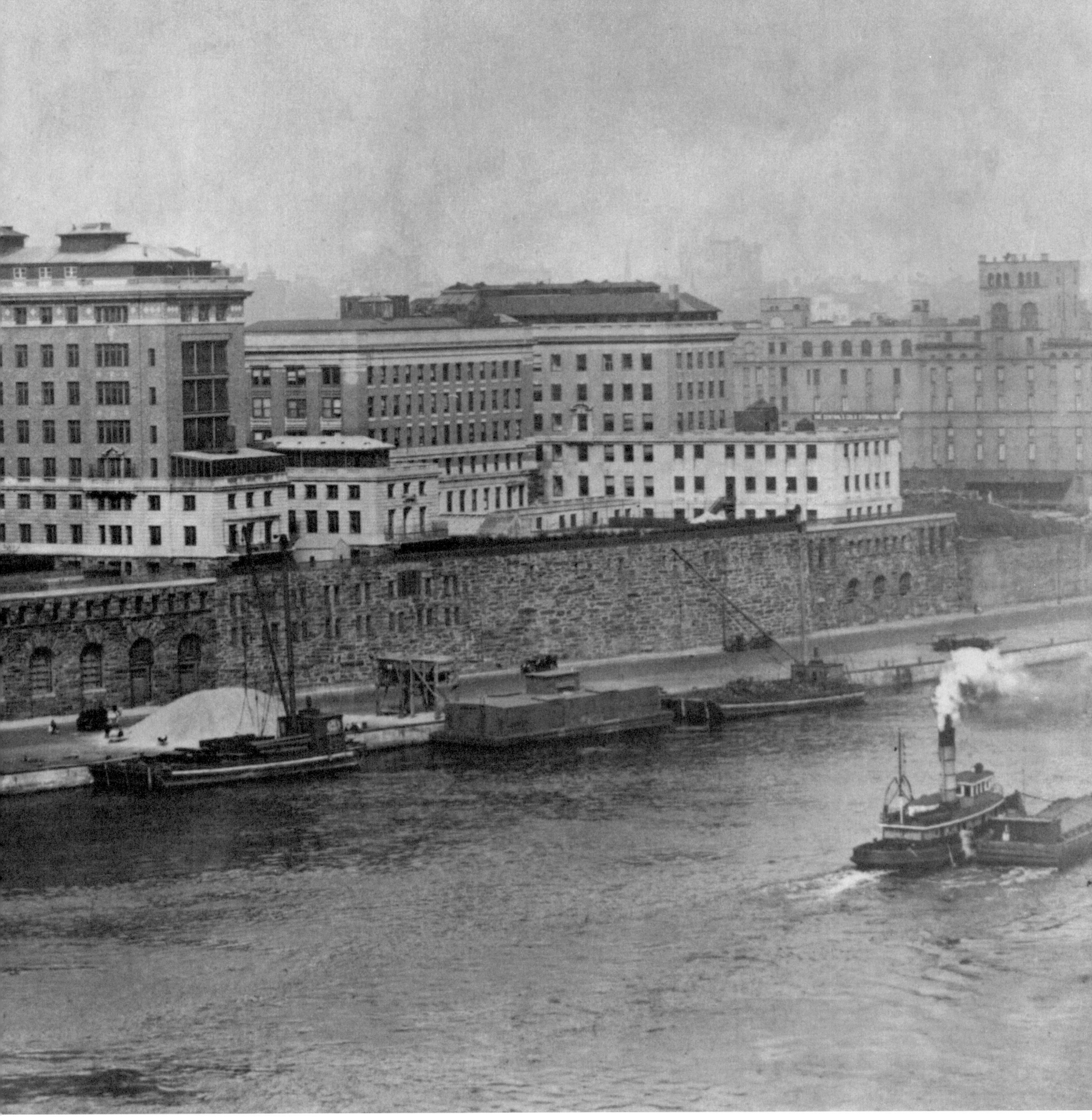

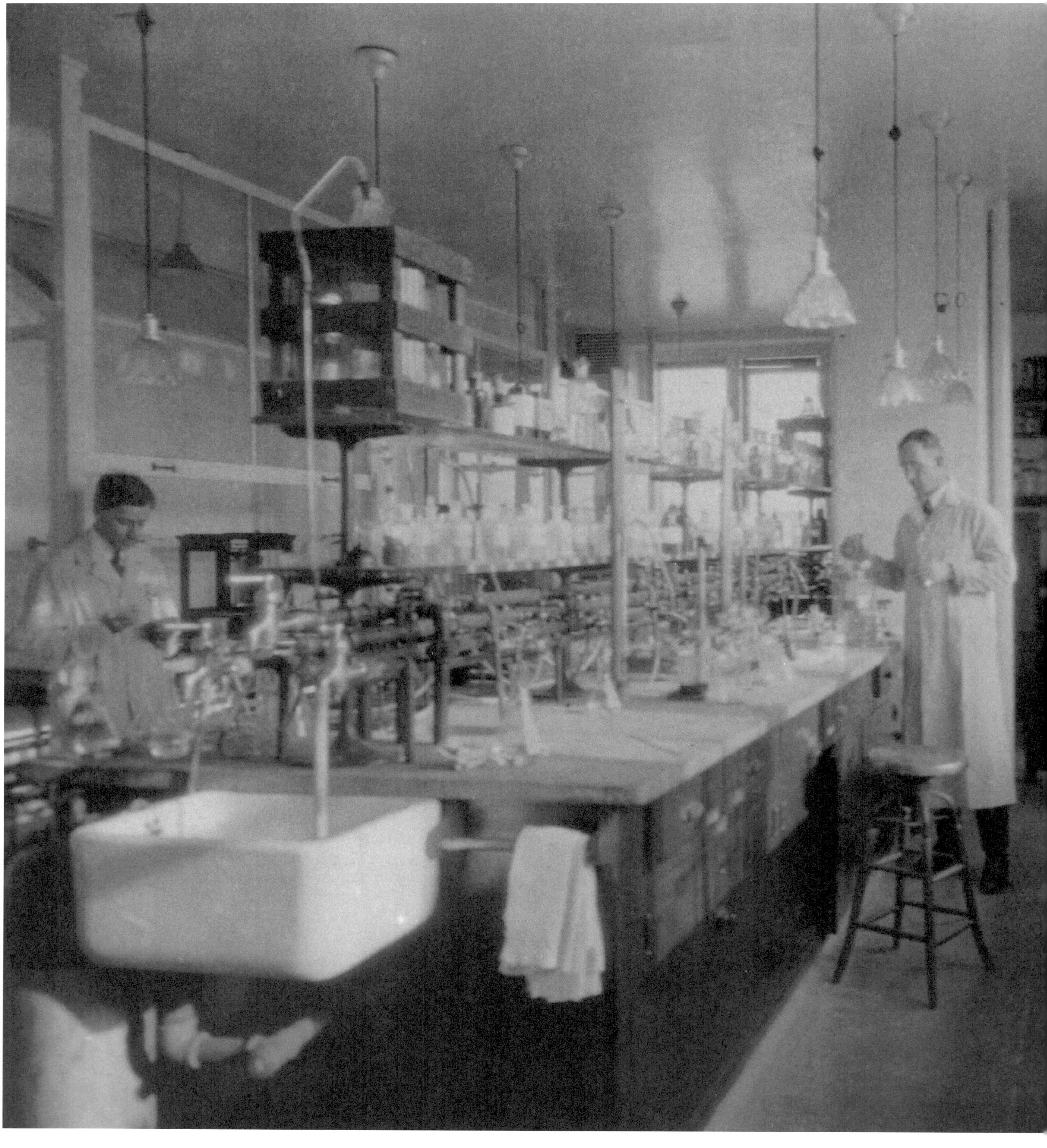

John D. Rockefeller Visits the Institute

John D. Rockefeller gave generously to The Rockefeller Institute but he stayed away from its affairs, relying on his son John D. Rockefeller Jr. and on Frederick Gates to keep him informed. For many years he declined even to visit the campus despite Simon Flexner's repeated invitations. "Very graciously he said that he could not take the valuable time of the workers," wrote Flexner. One day in the late 1920s, however, Rockefeller did visit. Walther F. Goebel, who came to the Institute in 1924, was among the scientists who spoke with him. Goebel, who died in 1993, gave this account in his unpublished memoir:

"Shortly after Michael [Heidelberger]'s departure, we had a distinguished visitor at the hospital. It was Mr. John D. Rockefeller, Senior, the founder of the institution which bore his name. A few days before his visit we had been told to make sure that our laboratories were orderly and clean. The windows on all eight floors of the hospital building glistened. The phalanx of Irish porters had long since polished all visible brass. Every nook and cranny was immaculate.

"Then, at mid-morning of the great day, Mr. Rockefeller's car, driven by a liveried chauffeur, arrived in front of our hospital. He was exposed to the elements, save for a black patent-leather awning. I believe the vehicle was known as a landaulet. One saw many in New York in those days. To own one was a badge of distinction.

"Mr. Rockefeller was greeted by Dr. Flexner and Dr. Cole. They then made their way to Dr. Cole's office on the seventh floor of the hospital. He spent a short while with Dr. Alfred Cohn. Then he visited Dr. Homer Swift and finally he had a short visit with Dr. Avery, who at the time was in the midst of his great discovery of the pneumococcal polysaccharides. To my surprise Dr. Avery brought Mr. Rockefeller upstairs to my laboratory—an unexpected visit that flustered me to no end.

I showed him samples of our extremely rare pneumococcal polysaccharides and quickly assembled the appropriate ingredients to demonstrate their remarkable property of serological specificity.

"As I recall, Mr. Rockefeller's visit was the last he made to our institution prior to his death a few years later. I remember him as an exceedingly alert, elderly gentleman who grasped the full implications of Dr. Avery's great discovery. As he left my laboratory he thanked me for my patience. He reached into his pocket, withdrew a coin, and presented me with one of his famous dimes, a symbol, no doubt, of his largesse."

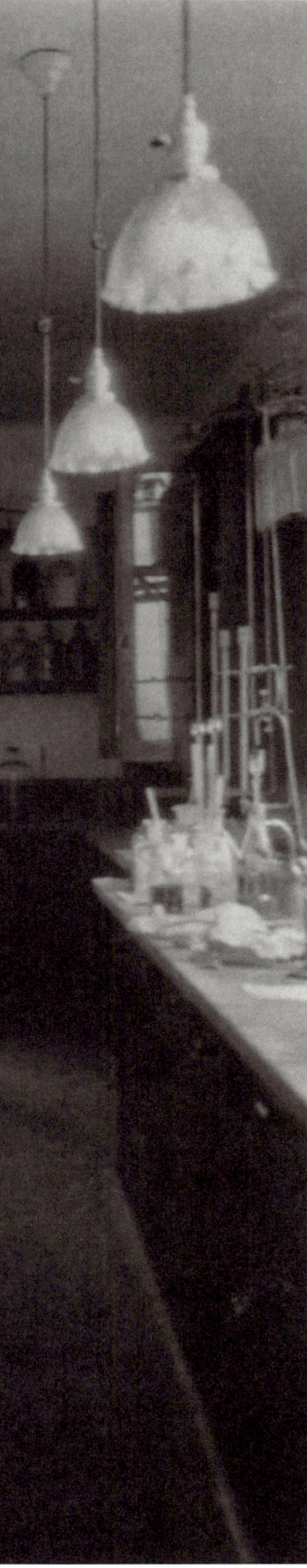

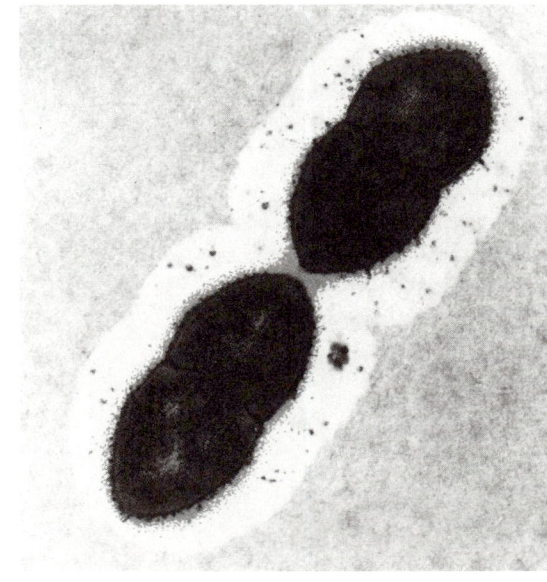

John D. Rockefeller visited laboratories in the Hospital similar to this one (left). Pneumococcus bacteria, the type studied by Oswald Avery, have a characteristic gelatinous coating (right).

Hidden Histories

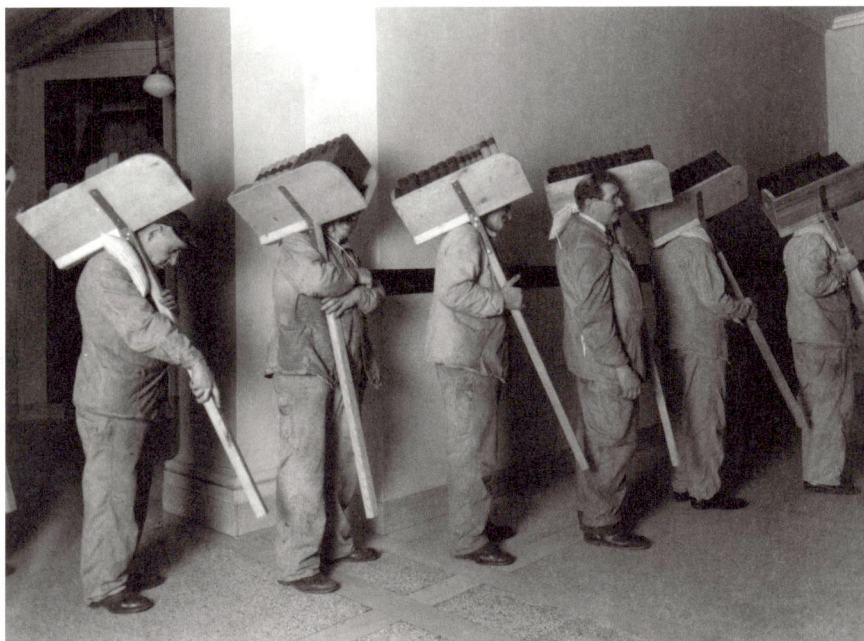

The achievements of Rockefeller's scientists are well known, but the work of the people who supported their science on a day-to-day basis—maintenance staff, workers in the laundry, technical assistants, hospital nurses, machinists in the instrument shop—remains largely hidden from history.

Simon Flexner took the same care in assembling a support staff for the Institute as he did in hiring scientists, recognizing their importance to scientific work. As Flexner put it, "There is no greater economy possible in laboratory organization than is to be derived from competent and well-trained" staff.

The histories of women who held research positions in the laboratories also remain unwritten. Only one woman—Florence Sabin—became a member, or full professor, in the first half of the Institute's history. But in the period before the Second World War, more than 50 others contributed directly to science at the Institute.

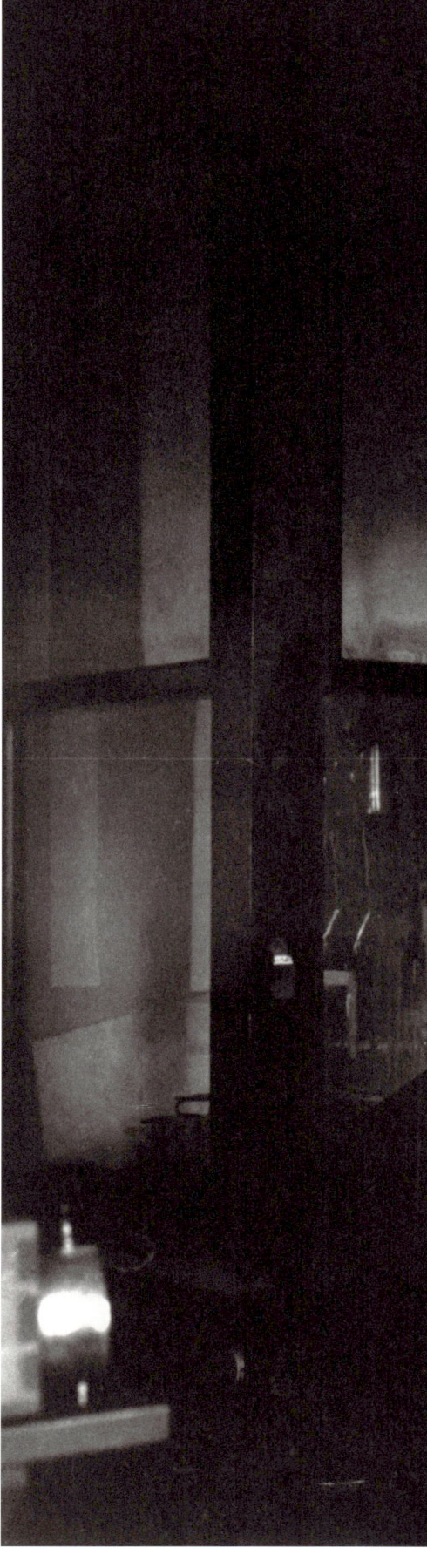

Workers move books into the new library in Welch Hall using bricklayers' hods. (1929) At right: Bertha Barker, a Wellesley graduate, had worked in a biology laboratory at M.I.T. before joining the laboratory of Eugene Opie in 1906. Alphonse Dochez is to her left.

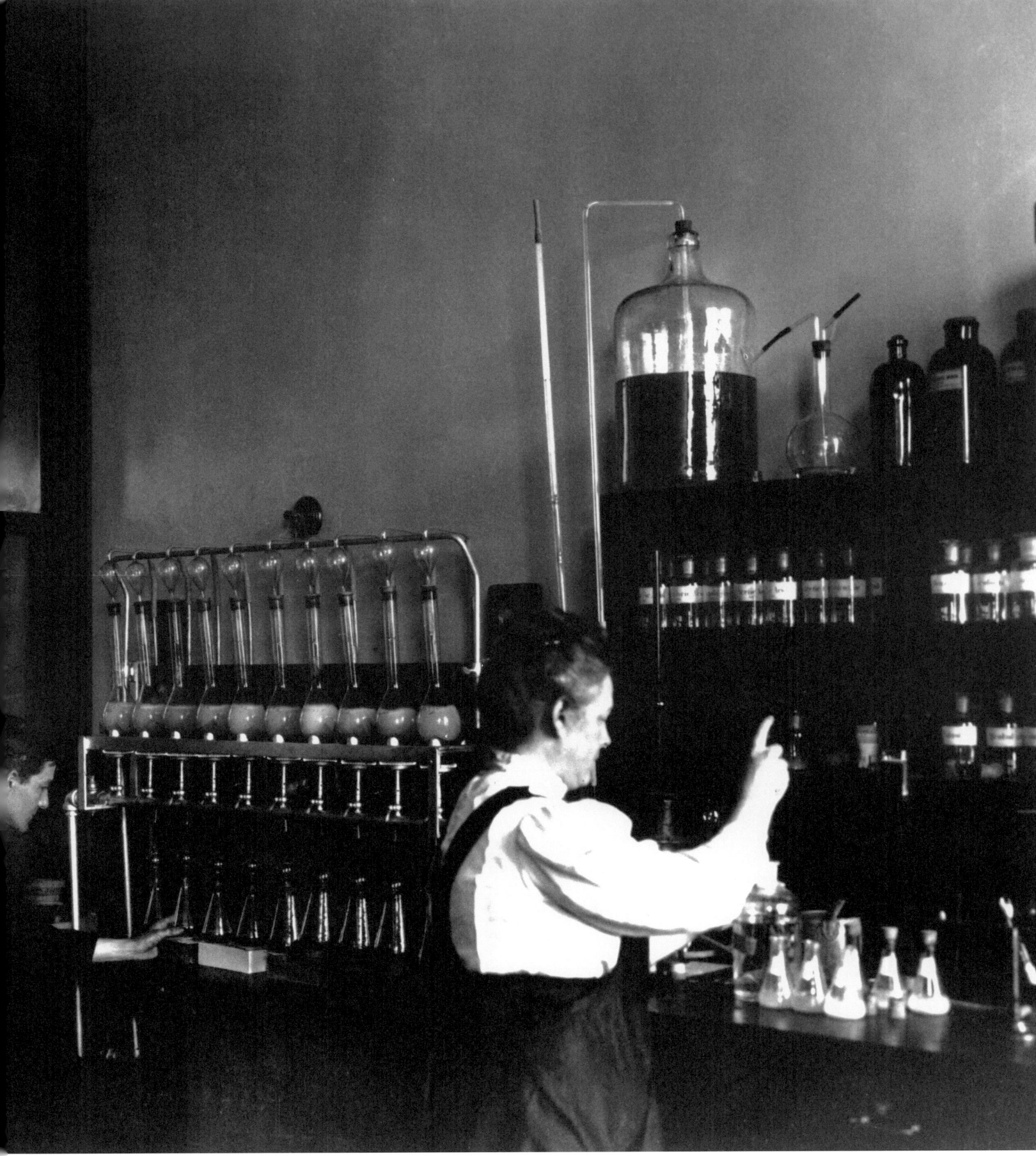

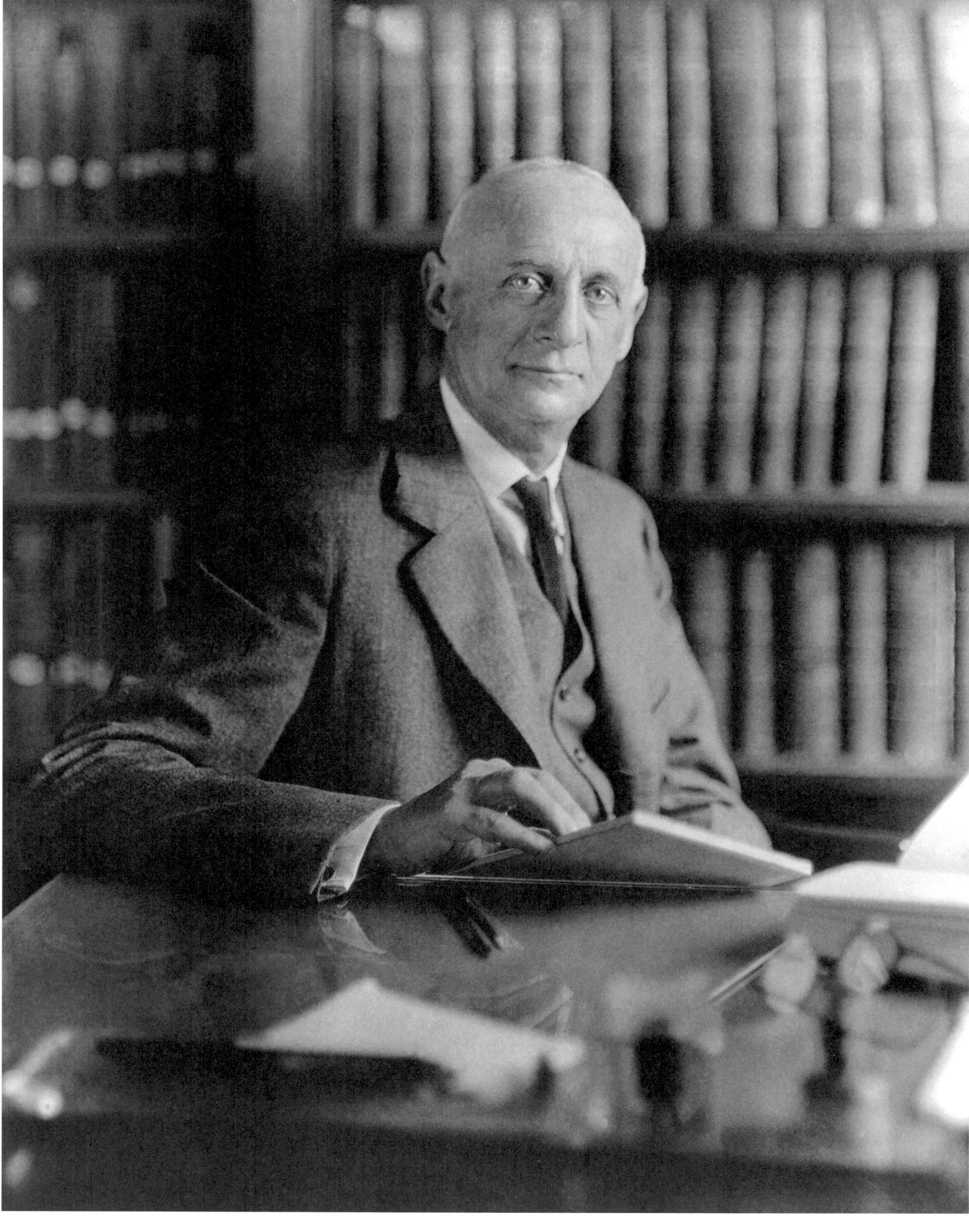

Simon Flexner

Simon Flexner is best remembered for his vision in creating The Rockefeller Institute for Medical Research and leading it for 33 years. But Flexner's contributions to the enterprise of research extended far beyond the Institute's boundaries. His position there allowed him to become a leader in scientific publishing, in communicating about science to the public, and in guiding the development of graduate and postgraduate science education in the United States and abroad.

Flexner recognized the importance of publishing the results of medical research. His mentor William H. Welch had founded *The Journal of Experimental Medicine* in 1896. But the work of editing the journal proved overwhelming for Welch, and by 1900 publication lapsed. In 1904 Flexner took over as editor and moved the journal to The Rockefeller Institute. He remained the journal's guiding force until his retirement.

As director of The Rockefeller Institute Flexner was a public figure, and he was called on to defend medical research in addition to promoting it. In the first decades of its history the Institute frequently came under attack by antivivisectionists. Flexner defended animal experimentation repeatedly, explaining its importance to newspaper reporters and fighting state legislation that would have limited research.

Although forced to take part in such public debates, Flexner more often worked behind the scenes to shape medical research. Education was as great a concern to him as it was to his brother Abraham Flexner, author of the 1910 report on medical education that resulted in the radical reform of American medical schools.

Rather than the training of M.D.'s, Simon Flexner's interest was in nurturing laboratory scientists who would focus on medical questions. He was a charter member of the Rockefeller Foundation and in this capacity he helped establish fellowships administered by the National Research Council that were vital in supplying opportunities for postdoctoral training for generations of American scientists. Detlev Bronk, later president of The Rockefeller University, was one of these fellows in the late 1920s. Flexner was also a trustee of the Carnegie Foundation and Johns Hopkins University.

Flexner retired quietly from his directorship of the Institute in 1935, but he continued to be a statesman for science. In 1937 and 1938 he was appointed Eastman Professor at Oxford University so that he could give advice as newly endowed medical professorships were organized there. As a result of this experience Flexner wrote a book, *The Evolution and Organization of the University Clinic*.

Although the Institute never granted degrees during his lifetime, Flexner's legacy—through the hundreds of scientists who gained research experience during temporary positions at the Institute and the recipients of the National Research Council's fellowships—may be considered largely educational. He was an extraordinary mentor with an uncommon ability for identifying talented researchers and drawing out their intellectual best.

Peyton Rous, who joined the Institute's staff in 1911, summed up Flexner's career this way: "During the fifty years of his personal effort medicine emerged into the sharp light of science. He helped this happen, and he did vastly more. He revealed the existence in the unconsidered human commonality of latent abilities to discover, and he showed that these could be called forth by fostering individual initiative and giving it scope. The planners of the Rockefeller Institute had thought of it as a purposeful utilization of human strength; but they had not known how to come at the strength, much less how to bring it to bear. Flexner did both."

Simon Flexner nurtured the careers of hundreds of medical researchers.

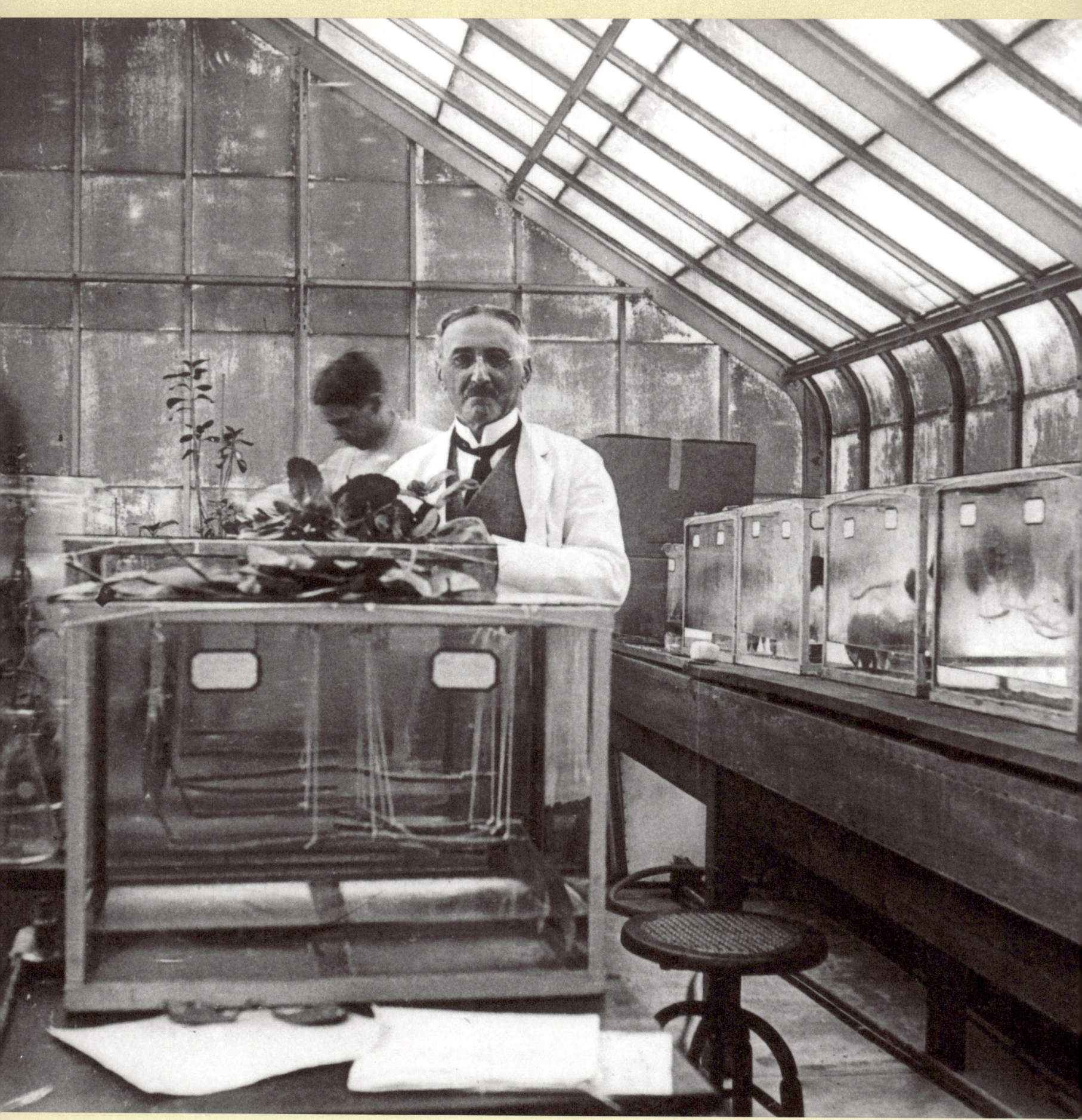

Jacques Loeb, the outspoken experimentalist, in an undated snapshot.

A VISION

Part 2: Medical Research Embraces the Physical Sciences

Simon Flexner's broad view of medical science set The Rockefeller Institute on a course that proved productive long beyond his service as director. He encouraged scientific work at the boundaries between the life sciences and the physical sciences, and the application of the theory and techniques of chemistry to the problems of medical research. The resulting research has been acknowledged with many Nobel Prizes over the century. "A cunning and subtle chemistry and physics, as well as biology, presides over all the happenings which separate…health from…disease," Flexner wrote. "Medical research, the most comprehensive perhaps of all kinds of research, requires, therefore, the employment of the knowledge and the methods of the biologist, chemist, and physicist."

Flexner, who came of age scientifically at a time when bacteriology epitomized medical research, traveled to Europe in 1903 and 1904 to learn firsthand the latest methods in chemistry. The trip also happened to be his honeymoon—he had married Helen Thomas in September 1903. Flexner took the opportunity to spend time at the Pasteur Institute and in the laboratory of the eminent chemist Emil Fischer, in Berlin.

When Flexner returned to New York, he appointed researchers to the Institute's faculty who stretched conventional notions of the boundaries of medical research. Jacques Loeb was particularly controversial. Loeb espoused a rigorously experimental approach to biology and mechanistic explanations of life processes. He was famous for experiments with sea urchin eggs—he had taken unfertilized sea urchin eggs and induced them to divide and begin to develop into larvae by changing the salt concentration of their water baths or by treating them with a chemical. The action of sperm in the fundamental process of fertilization could thus be understood as a chemical switch that triggered the dormant potential of the egg to develop. From this and work with other lower animals, Loeb concluded that "all life phenomena" might be explained solely in terms of chemical mechanisms.

Flexner invited Loeb to join the faculty in 1909, and some Board members and others at the Institute challenged his choice. What did experiments with sea urchins and worms have to do with the complexities of human health and disease, they asked. Loeb's approach to biology was far from medical research as traditionally construed—anatomy, pathology, physiology, and pharmacology. Loeb himself responded to these doubts. "In my opinion experimental biology—the experimental biology of the cell—will have to form the basis not only of physiology but also of general pathology and therapeutics. I do not think that the medical schools in this country are ready for the new departure…. The only place in America where such a new departure could be made for the cause of medicine would be The Rockefeller Institute or an institution with similar tendencies. The medical public at large does not yet fully see the bearing of the new science of experimental biology (in the sense in which I understand it) on medicine."

Loeb's appointment as a member of the Institute in 1910 illustrated Flexner's broadminded commitment to bold approaches to the study of disease, and Loeb's views set the tone for inquiry at Rockefeller. Loeb taunted the M.D.'s at the Institute at a time when medicine was widely criticized as lacking rigor. "Medical science?" he asked. "That is a contradiction in terms. There is no such thing." The criticism stung. Alfred E. Cohn, who became head of cardiology at the Hospital, recalled that "Loeb, the most accomplished, the most intelligent, and, we thought, the wisest man with whom it was our privilege to come in contact, as we did daily in our lunch room, we thought was laughing at us."

Some physicians may have felt insecure when faced with such a forceful personality as Loeb. But clinical research at the Rockefeller Hospital embraced the physical sciences from the beginning. Rufus Cole, the Hospital director, believed that Hospital research aimed at understanding the underlying causes of a disease should entail much more than a detailed description of the course of the illness. Rather, clinical investigation required physicians who were also skilled in the laboratory. Both bedside observation and laboratory work were needed to get at the roots of an ailment. Indeed, many M.D. members of the Institute (the equivalent of full professors) were elected to the National Academy of Sciences, testament to their accomplishments in the laboratory.

The University of Michigan tried to recruit Rufus Cole, but he accepted the position of director of The Rockefeller Institute Hospital instead.

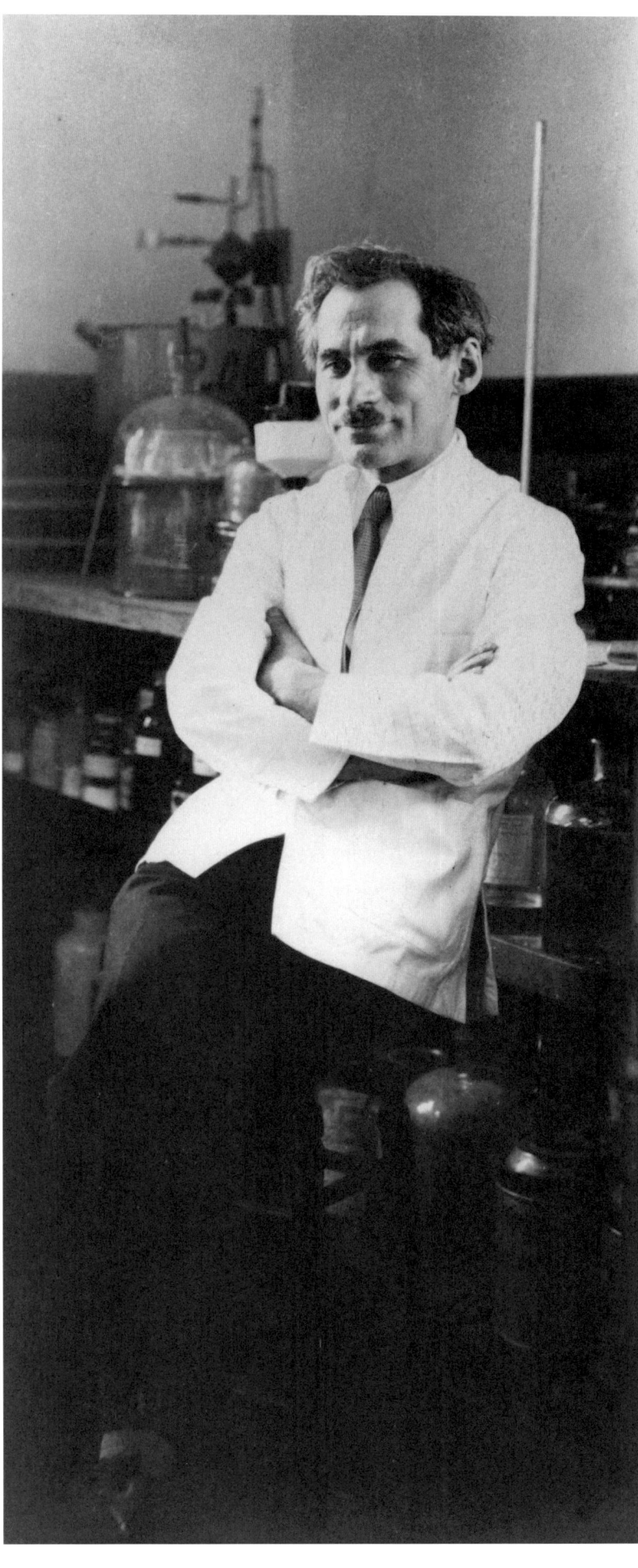

Chemist Phoebus A.T. Levene was one of the first scientists Simon Flexner hired for the Institute. In 1907 Levene wrote to Board member L. Emmett Holt, "I have received your communication of my election Member of the Institute. I can think of no greater honor…"

In 1909, as the Hospital was being built, Cole spent a year honing his own bench skills in the chemistry laboratory of P.A.T. Levene. Levene was well established in his field when he arrived at Rockefeller in 1905, and he worked 35 years at the Institute pioneering chemical knowledge of biologically important molecules, most famously nucleic acids. Levene identified the key components of DNA and RNA, molecules that were known to be significant although their roles in heredity had not yet been discovered. Working with Levene was a young chemist named Donald D. Van Slyke, who would become one of the first success stories in Cole's efforts to establish a new style of clinical investigation at Rockefeller. Cole met Van Slyke during his year of work in Levene's laboratory, and in 1914 Van Slyke moved over to the Hospital staff.

Van Slyke, a founder of clinical chemistry, is widely remembered for the apparatus he developed around 1920 to measure oxygen and carbon dioxide in blood. Chemical analysis of blood samples in order to diagnose disease—so routine today as to be unremarkable—was then a new idea. But bringing the methods of chemistry to clinical diagnosis required first inventing the means for measuring gases and other substances in the blood. With his device, Van Slyke identified blood abnormalities that diagnosed diabetes and discovered that influenza patients often died from a lack of oxygen in their blood—in effect, they suffocated. For the first time doctors understood the reasons that oxygen therapy helped flu patients. Van Slyke's interest in quantifying blood gases, as well as substances in other body fluids, led him to study the changes in metabolism, blood chemistry, and urine excretion that characterize kidney diseases. Although he was a Ph.D. chemist and not an M.D., he oversaw the care of hundreds of kidney patients at the Rockefeller Hospital until his retirement in 1948.

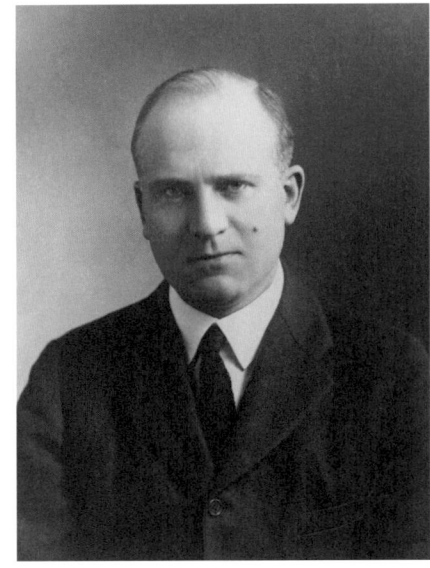

Donald D. Van Slyke invented instruments for analyzing blood chemistry.

Discovering DNA

At the same time that Van Slyke was making such progress in quantifying clinical diagnoses, Oswald T. Avery led a quiet revolution in another Hospital laboratory that would forever change biology and the way the world thought about heredity. His most important discovery—that DNA is the carrier of hereditary information—was the result of more than 20 years of painstaking study. It was a finding that demonstrated the success of Simon Flexner's founding philosophy of allowing researchers the freedom and resources to pursue long-term studies.

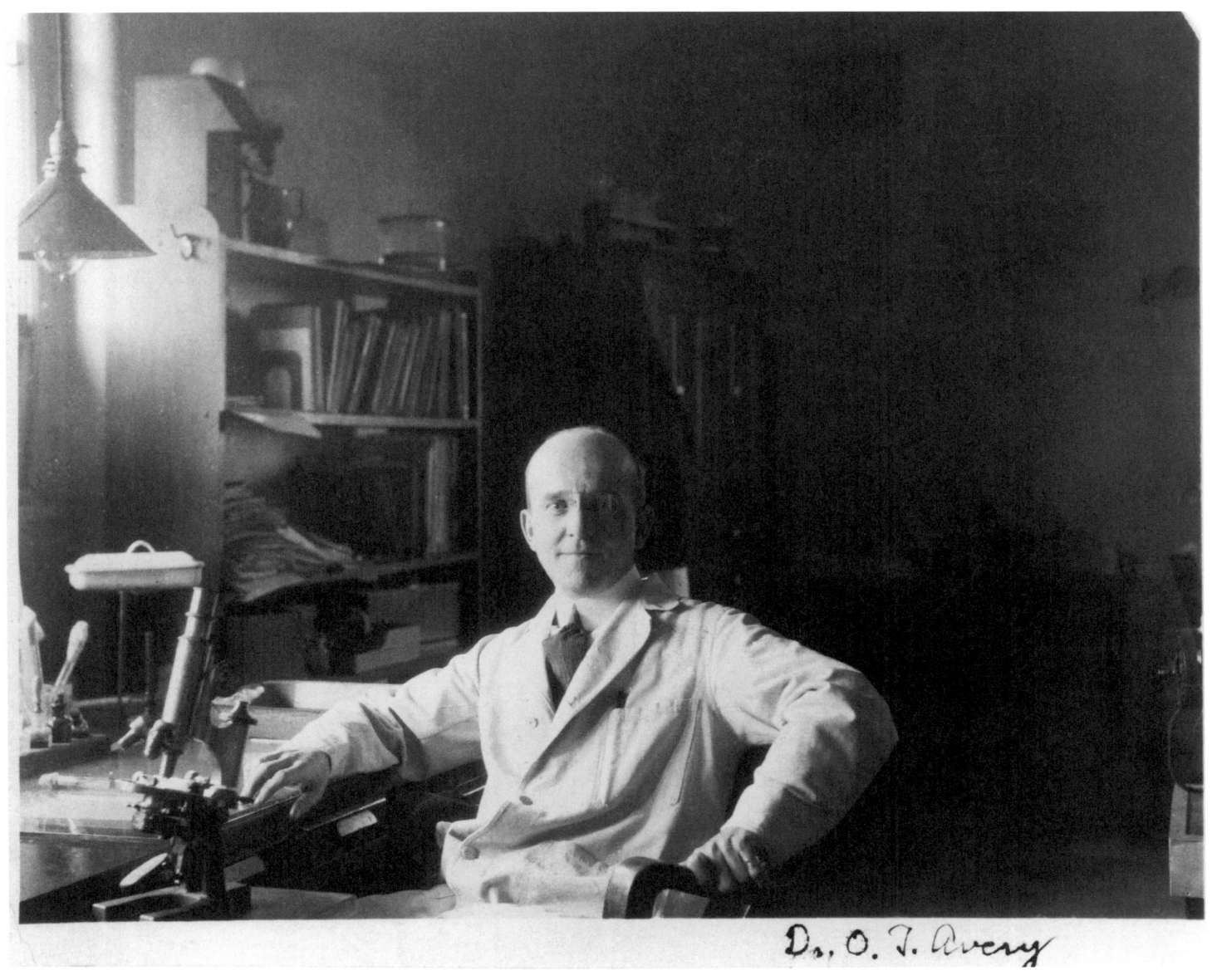

Oswald T. Avery devoted his career to studying pneumococcus, a bacterium that causes pneumonia.

Rufus Cole recruited Avery to Rockefeller in 1913 to find a way to treat pneumococcal pneumonia. At the beginning of the 20th century this type of pneumonia killed more than 20 percent of those infected—50,000 people per year in the United States. So severe was its impact that the great physician William Osler called pneumonia "captain of the men of death," a phrase that in earlier years had been applied to tuberculosis. Avery's own mother had died of the disease. Understanding the cause of pneumonia and finding a cure were high priorities for the Rockefeller Hospital.

Before Avery joined the staff, Cole himself had attempted to develop a therapeutic serum against pneumonia. Similar serums—crude sorts of after-the-fact vaccines— had been somewhat successful in treating diphtheria and cerebrospinal meningitis. However, Cole and his coworkers soon discovered that there were several strains of pneumococcal bacteria, and some were more virulent than others. By the cumbersome methods of the day, each would require treatment with a different serum. Progress depended on understanding the slight chemical differences among the various strains.

Avery and his coworkers continued the work and discovered that the secret to the bacterium's virulence lay in an unusual feature: under the microscope, they could see that pneumococcus bacteria are enveloped in a gelatinous coating, or capsule. This capsule protects the bacteria from the immune defenses of the organism they have infected. When scientists removed the capsule from bacteria grown in petri dishes, the bacteria were no longer virulent. Avery and his colleagues made advances in diagnosing the type of pneumococcal bacteria that infected patients and continued work on antibacterial serums. But to devise a therapy, they needed to understand the chemical nature of the capsule.

What transpired next exemplified the kind of cross-disciplinary synthesis that Flexner hoped to nurture by having physicians, biologists, chemists, and physicists working on medical research in the same small institution. Avery enlisted the chemist Michael Heidelberger, who was working in Van Slyke's laboratory, to help with the pneumococcus problem. Together with others in Avery's lab, they broke down the capsule into its constituent chemical parts and tested each for the immunological reaction it provoked in laboratory mice.

This led, in 1923, to the first of Avery's great discoveries: that the pneumococcus capsule was made up of complexly linked sugar molecules. This finding flew in the face of conventional wisdom, which held that only protein molecules could stimulate an immune reaction. The specific virulence of a pneumococcal strain depended on which sugars made up its capsule.

An "extracurricular" experiment started by René Dubos in Avery's laboratory led to the first systematic discovery of an antibiotic. This page from the 1939 notebook of Rollin Hotchkiss, who worked with Dubos, shows steps in the purification of the antibiotic, which was at first called gramidinic acid.

Dubos and Hotchkiss went on to head their own laboratories at Rockefeller. The work of Hotchkiss, and of Norton Zinder, who joined him in 1952, furthered knowledge of the mechanisms of heredity and of bacterial resistance to antibiotics.

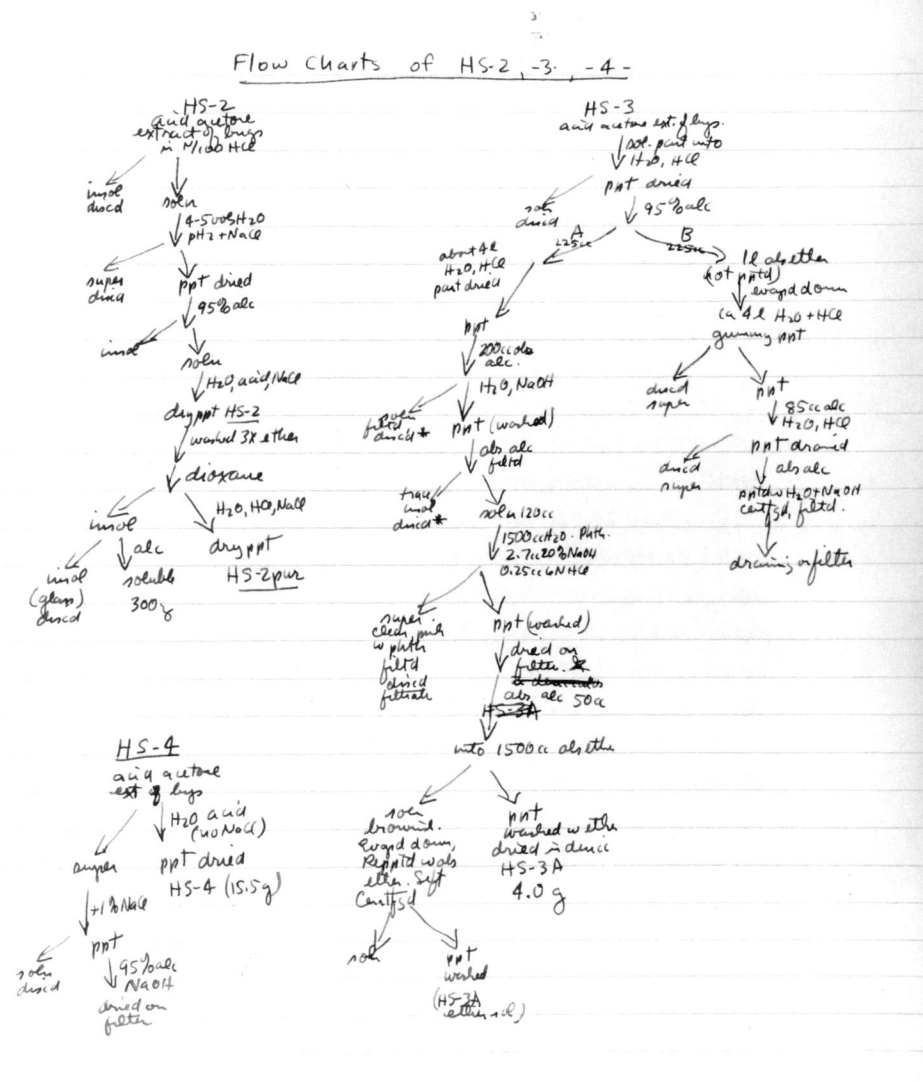

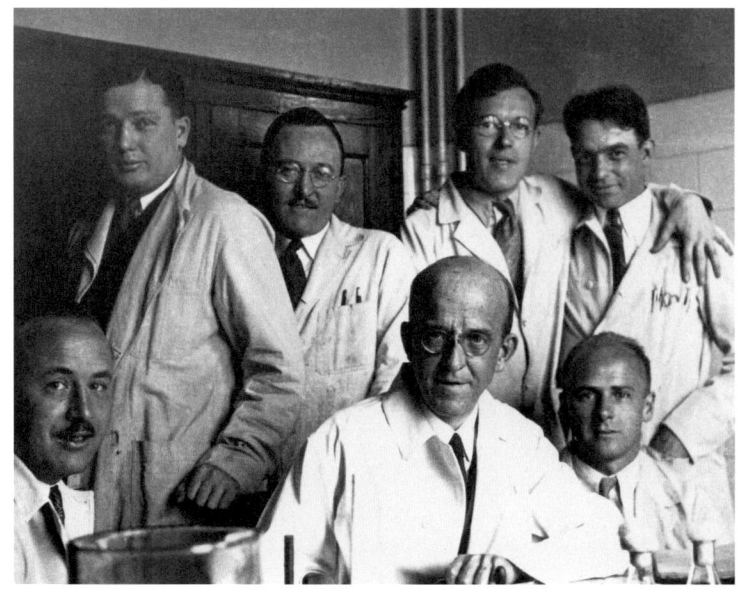

Scientists in Oswald Avery's laboratory in the early 1930s included (left to right): seated, Thomas Francis Jr., Avery, Walther F. Goebel; standing, Edward E. Terrell, Kenneth Goodner, René J. Dubos, and Frank H. Babers.

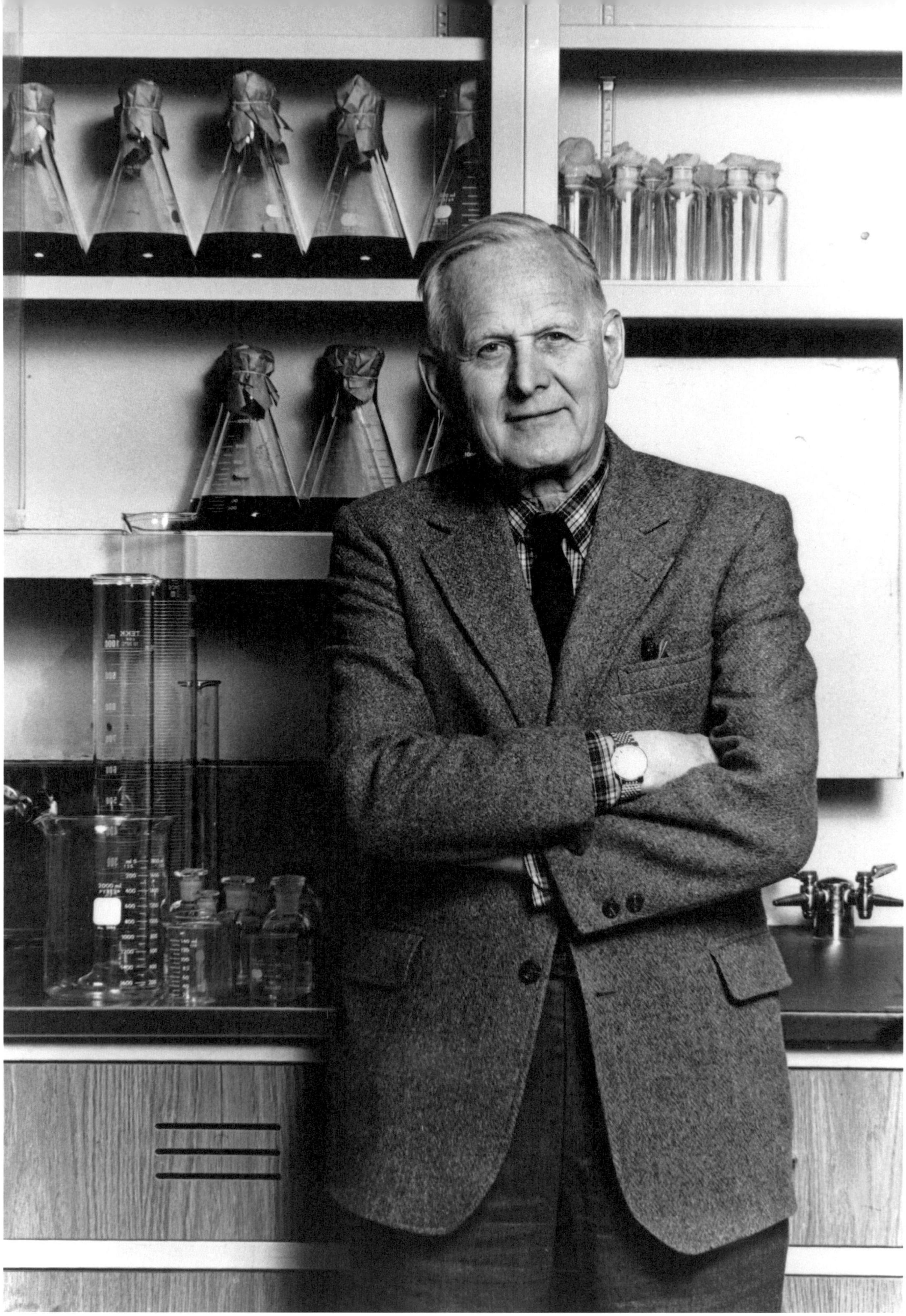

Maclyn McCarty collaborated with Oswald Avery and Colin MacLeod on the landmark experiments showing that DNA carries hereditary information. McCarty, who joined Avery's laboratory in 1941, was physician-in-chief of the Hospital from 1960 to 1974 and vice president of the University from 1965 to 1978.

The finding for which Avery is most remembered was another two decades in the making, and it, too, challenged scientific orthodoxy. In 1928 the British researcher Frederick Griffith described a phenomenon called "transformation." Under certain circumstances, pneumococcus bacteria that had been stripped of their capsules could be induced to switch types—to transform into a different type of pneumococcus, with a capsule.

Griffith's experiment had been to infect laboratory mice with two kinds of harmless pneumococcal bacteria simultaneously. One type was live but crippled—it had lost its ability to make a capsule, and thus would be killed by mouse immune defenses. The other type was whole, but had been killed by heat. Individually, neither type should have harmed the mice. But Griffith's mice, infected with both types, died from an infection of living, virulent bacteria of the type that had been injected dead. Somehow, the living, capsule-less bacteria had been transformed into a virulent encapsulated type. Taking up this problem, Avery and his colleagues established that the dead bacteria had transferred an unknown chemical to the capsule-less cells. This substance enabled them to grow capsules and evade the mouse immune system.

Again, Avery focused on the chemistry of the problem. What was the chemical nature of this so-called transforming agent? With his young colleagues Colin M. MacLeod and Maclyn McCarty, overcoming daunting technical difficulties and his own illness with Graves' disease, Avery identified the substance as DNA. As the group prepared to publish its results, which appeared in 1944, Avery wrote to his brother, a bacteriologist at Vanderbilt University: "Try to find in that complex mixture the active principle!! Try to isolate and chemically identify the particular substance that will by itself when brought into contact with the R cell derived from Type II cause it to elaborate Type III capsular polysaccharide, and to acquire all the aristocratic distinctions of the same specific type of cells as that from which the extract was prepared! Some job—and full of heartaches and heartbreaks. But at last *perhaps* we have it."

The DNA discovery launched the era of molecular biology by laying the groundwork for understanding the structure and function of the molecules of heredity. Like so many research successes at Rockefeller, it began with scientists asking fundamental questions about the nature of disease. Questions aimed initially at improving treatment for pneumonia led to an even more significant achievement. At the same time, the search for a pneumonia cure was never abandoned; but just as Avery's research group was close to finding a new therapy, antibiotics became available for treating the disease and its reputation as a killer receded.

A View Into the Cell

Just a year after Avery and his coworkers announced their discovery of the hereditary importance of the DNA molecule, another group of Rockefeller researchers published a paper that opened the way to a new understanding of the cell. Like the DNA work, it began with an investigation into a disease—in this case cancer—and brought together an interdisciplinary team of researchers who applied quantitative and chemical techniques to a stubborn biological problem.

Every basic biology textbook contains a now-familiar, stylized illustration of a cell. Inside the cell membrane are the nucleus, the mitochondria, the endoplasmic reticulum, the lysosome, and other organelles that carry out the functions that keep the cell alive. Although this knowledge is taken for granted today, the cell's interior was unmapped territory until the 1940s, in part because the low resolution of light microscopes allowed scientists to see only a disorganized blur inside cells. In the 1930s and 1940s a group of researchers working in the Rockefeller laboratory of James B. Murphy brought that view into focus for the first time.

Albert Claude had come to Rockefeller in 1929 to try to isolate the agent known to cause a transmissible form of cancer in chickens, today called the Rous sarcoma virus. To do this he perfected ways of separating the components of cells using a centrifuge; he spun the cell cultures at rates as high as 18,000 rpm, forcing their components to settle in layers of different weights, called fractions. He not only was able to purify the tumor-causing agent but he also found, in all the cell types he examined, something that he called a microsome. The microsome seemed to be essential to cells, yet it was too tiny to see with a standard light microscope.

Claude's 1943 paper describing microsomes prompted a phone call from the director of the research laboratories of the Interchemical Corporation in New York. That company, as it happened, possessed an electron microscope, a new type of instrument that was capable of imaging structures 100 times smaller than those visible through a light microscope. A collaboration ensued between Claude and Ernest Fullam, the microscopist at the company, to analyze fractions containing cell components such as microsomes.

In addition to looking at microsomes alone, Claude and Fullam wanted to see where the microsomes were located in whole, intact cells. To view whole cells they sought the help of Keith Porter, a zoologist who came to work in Murphy's lab in 1939.

Albert Claude helped launch the modern science of cell biology, research honored in 1974 with a Nobel Prize shared with George Palade and Christian de Duve. (1940s)

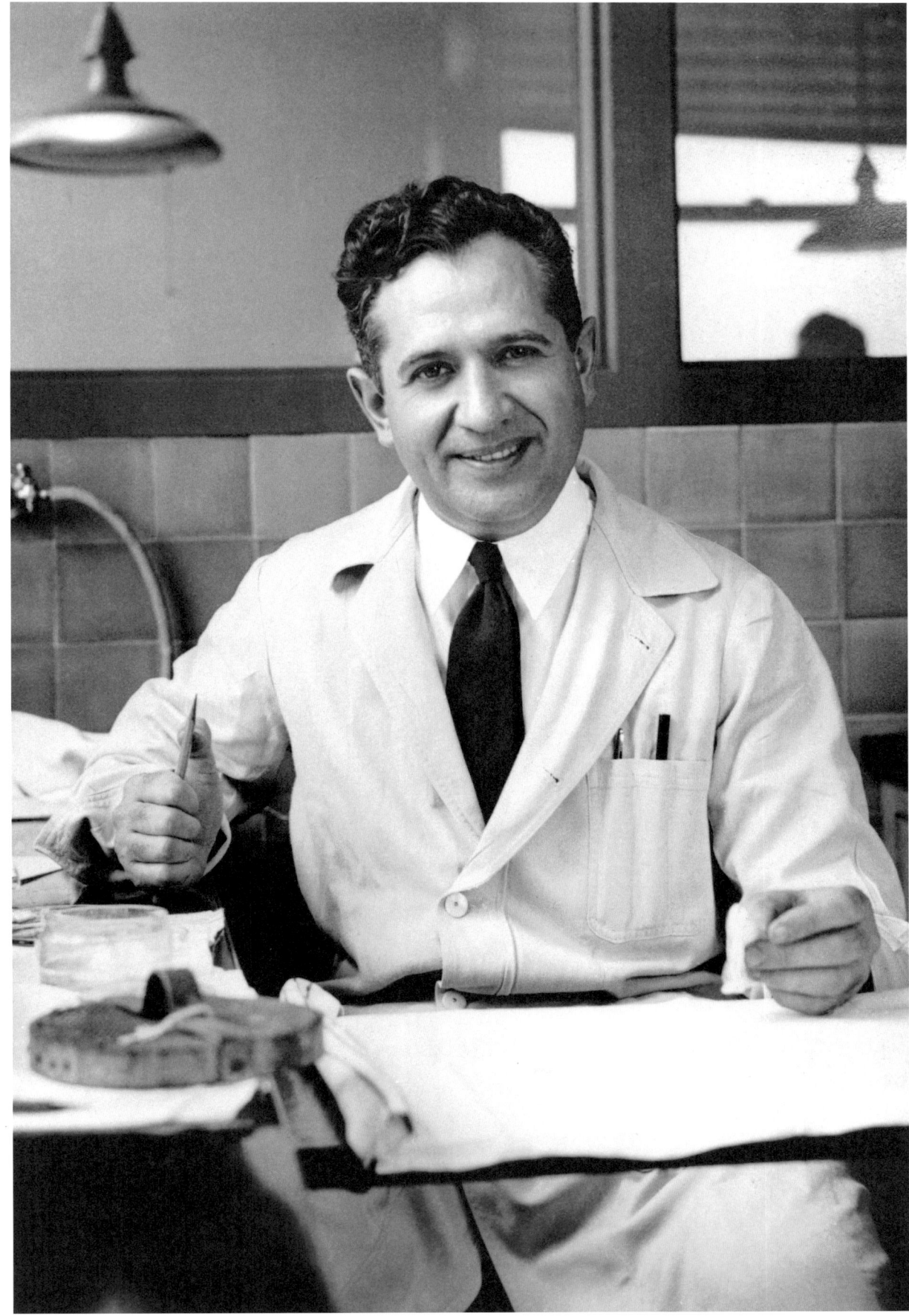

61

Porter was an expert in cell culture, the art of growing cells in petri dishes. To see cells with the electron microscope, the researchers needed a sheet of cells grown in a layer only one cell thick. Besides achieving this technical feat, Porter also had to devise a way of drying and chemically stabilizing the cells without distorting their structure; he knew from experience that preparing cells for microscope viewing often changed their shape.

Finally, in 1944, the pooled expertise of these three researchers resulted in the first image of an intact cell—a connective tissue cell from a chicken embryo—at a resolution that revealed a new landscape of structures inside. Before the electron microscope, Claude recalled, biologists had been "in the same situation as astronomers and astrophysicists, who were permitted to see the objects of their interest, but not to touch them; the cell was as distant from us as the stars and galaxies were from them."

The collaborative work at Rockefeller gave rise to a new understanding of the structure and function of cells. In the decades since, the field of cell biology has maintained a strong base at Rockefeller. George Palade came to Rockefeller in 1946 and perfected electron microscopy in the course of discovering the functions of individual cell components during various stages of cell growth. In 1962, Christian de Duve joined the Rockefeller faculty. Among other achievements he had discovered the lysosome, a cell organelle responsible for waste disposal. Claude, de Duve, and Palade were awarded a Nobel Prize in 1974 for discoveries concerning the functional organization of the cell. The distinguished lineage of cell biologists at Rockefeller continues today, and was acknowledged in 1999 by another Nobel Prize. This one was awarded to Günter Blobel, who joined the laboratory of Palade and Philip Siekevitz in 1967 and, in turn, has trained a new generation of cell biologists.

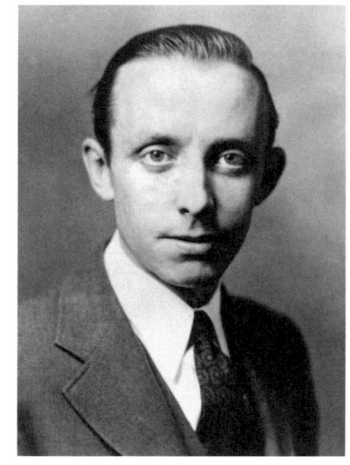

Keith Porter developed techniques for growing cells so that they could be imaged with the electron microscope.

George Palade (left) explored the cell interior, discovering previously unknown structures and their functions. He shared a 1974 Nobel Prize with Albert Claude and Christian de Duve.

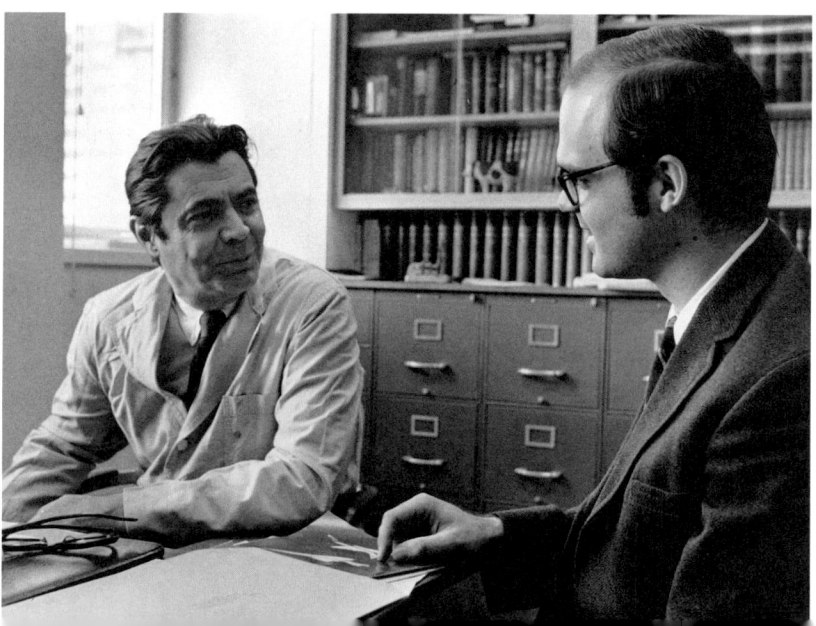

This electron micrograph was the first to show an intact cell. The cell was a fibroblast—a cell that gives rise to connective tissue—taken from a chicken embryo.

A Golden Age for Science

The discovery of DNA's significance and the founding of the field of cell biology are perhaps the two achievements for which Rockefeller is most famous, but the Institute's first half-century was an extraordinarily productive time in many other areas. Rockefeller was a leading center for research on viruses and tissue culture, the technique of keeping cells and tissues alive in the artificial environment of petri dishes and laboratory flasks. Pioneering studies of infectious diseases such as rheumatic fever and tuberculosis continued. And the flip side of infection—immunology—became an important focus of research.

The Rockefeller Institute for Medical Research remained a fairly small institution. Between 1930 and 1950 the number of laboratories it supported hovered around 20. This number was small enough so that the scientists and their associates met every day for lunch in Welch dining hall, an occasion that constituted an intensive year-round seminar. They were, in the words of Paul de Kruif, a "bevy of bacteriological, biological big names."

As the leading biomedical research institute in the country, Rockefeller attracted top talent, both locally and internationally. At mid-century the director of the Institute could choose from a much larger population of highly trained scientists than at the Institute's founding, and no longer did he have trouble convincing them to come to Rockefeller. The Institute's researchers were prominent members of national and international scientific and policy organizations. To a large extent this success and the key to the Institute's scientific productivity lay in Simon Flexner's broad-minded approach to the study of disease and the consistency of his vision of the laboratory as a stand-alone element, a legacy that lives on today.

Flexner retired as director in 1935. His successor, Herbert Gasser, shepherded the work at Rockefeller along much the same trajectory that Flexner had started. Gasser was a physiologist, known for his studies of the conduction of nerve impulses, for which he received a Nobel Prize in 1944. He inherited a well-managed, productive institution and endeavored to maintain its reputation for excellence. Gasser broadened the fields of research of the Institute, bringing in a group of biophysicists and boosting resources for the study of proteins by physical and chemical methods. Under his leadership, the Board of Scientific Directors also shifted from a majority of medical doctors to a group more broadly representative of the Institute's research, including men trained in other fields of science.

The 1930s Intellectual Migration

Max Bergmann was one of tens of thousands of European intellectuals, many of them Jewish, who came to the United States in the 1930s to escape fascist governments. A chemist, Bergmann emigrated from Germany in 1934, the year after Hitler rose to power and began dismissing thousands of university faculty and leaders of government cultural organizations. Bergmann had been forced to "retire" from the directorship of the Kaiser Wilhelm Institute for Leather Research in Dresden, a prestigious center for chemistry research. Simon Flexner facilitated Bergmann's immigration and appointed him a Member of the Institute. At Rockefeller Bergmann assembled a remarkable group of young physical chemists, two of whom—Stanford Moore and William Stein—went on to win Nobel Prizes.

February 24, 1934.

Dear Sir:

I am writing to ask your advice regarding the possibility of having Professor Max Bergmann and his wife admitted to this country, in order that Professor Bergmann may accept an appointment to the Scientific Staff of the Rockefeller Institute.

Professor Bergmann and Mrs. Bergmann were admitted to this country on November 6, 1933 as nonimmigrants, Class 2 of Section 3, of the Immigration Act of 1924, for a period of six months. Professor Bergmann came to the United States for the purpose of lecturing at various institutions and universities in this country. At the expiration of his initial period of admission his time of temporary stay was extended to June 20, 1934, in order to permit him to accept invitations to give additional lectures.

The Rockefeller Institute now desires to offer Professor Bergmann an appointment as Associate on its Scientific Staff. Under the Institute's rules an appointment as Associate can be for a period of three years only. Although no assurance can be given that Professor Bergmann's appointment will be continued, nevertheless I would say that appointments as Associate are rarely made except with the expectation that the Institute will find it desirable to offer its facilities for more than three years.

As you may know Professor Bergmann is generally considered one of a relatively small group of outstanding German chemists. If he is permitted to accept this appointment he will bring to the Institute an experience and training in his special field which is unique. For this reason the Institute does not feel that in offering this appointment to Professor Bergmann it will be replacing any person in this country. On the other hand, the setting up of a laboratory for Professor Bergmann will permit the Institute to engage several assistants highly trained in chemistry, as well as a number of technical helpers. Hence, positions will be created which would otherwise remain unfilled.

Under normal conditions it would be suggested to Professor Bergmann that he return to Germany and apply to an American Consulate General there for permission to enter this country as a "professor", for which classification he would be eligible by reason of his recent experience. However, due to conditions in Germany, with which I am sure you are familiar, Professor Bergmann feels that serious obstacles to his return to the United States might be placed in his way by German authorities. I would, therefore, appreciate your opinion as to whether or not it would be in order to suggest to Professor Bergmann that he proceed to Canada and apply to an American Consulate General there for admission to this country as a "professor". If this seems advisable, may I ask you to inform me what documents, etc., the American Consulate to whom he applies will require in considering his application.

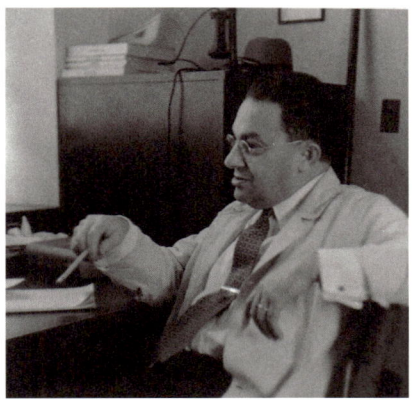

As the Nazis gained power in Germany in the 1930s, Jewish intellectuals fled the country. Many were scientists who came to the United States, including chemist Max Bergmann, who joined Rockefeller's faculty in 1934.

Science Publishing

When the first cell biologists at Rockefeller wanted to publish their results, they found that existing journals could not print high-quality reproductions of electron microscope images. Furthermore, the old journals often turned down their papers because editors did not recognize the significance of discoveries in the new field. So in 1955, led by Keith Porter and H. Stanley Bennett, a group of cell biologists founded *The Journal of Biophysical and Biochemical Cytology*, published by The Rockefeller Institute. In 1962 the name was changed to *The Journal of Cell Biology*.

The Institute had been in the business of science publishing since 1905, when it took over *The Journal of Experimental Medicine* under the editorship of Simon Flexner. In 1918 Jacques Loeb and W.J.V. Osterhout founded *The Journal of General Physiology* at the Institute. All three journals came under the management of The Rockefeller Institute Press when it was formed in 1958. At the same time, the Press—today The Rockefeller University Press—began publishing occasional books on subjects related to biomedical research.

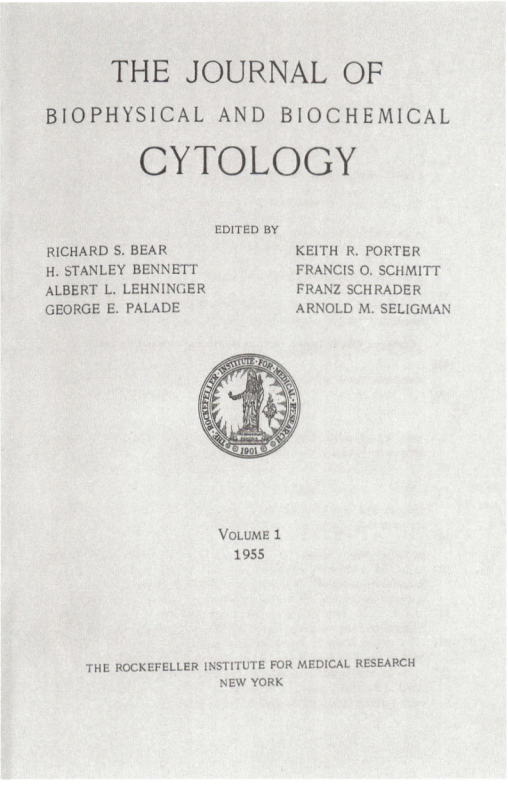

A VISION

A Closer Look: Medical Research Embraces the Physical Sciences

Food for Thinking 68

The Living Crystal 70

Karl Landsteiner 72

Herbert Gasser 75

Science and War 76

Tools for Discovery 79

Food for Thinking

Researchers who worked at Rockefeller through the 1960s recall a daily lunch hour charged with shop talk and camaraderie. The atmosphere was formal: table service, linen cloths, and fresh French bread. Laboratory groups generally sat together, and from the heads of the tables set for eight, senior faculty led freewheeling discussions of work in progress, tutored their younger colleagues, and entertained guests.

One of those visitors, in 1927, was René Dubos, then a young soil bacteriologist just completing a fellowship at Rutgers University. He had come to Rockefeller to pay a visit to fellow Frenchman Alexis Carrel. At lunch, Carrel seated Dubos next to Oswald Avery, who was at the time attempting to produce a serum for treating deadly lobar pneumonia. At the heart of the problem was finding a substance that was harmless to people but toxic to pneumonia bacteria—something that would destroy the capsule that surrounds each bacterium.

Dubos told Avery he could solve this problem by finding a microbe that would digest the capsule. Then he would extract the microbe's digestive enzyme. Impressed with this young man's confidence, Avery offered Dubos a fellowship and thus launched an investigation that would lead to the first systematic discovery of an antibiotic.

Dubos later attributed his success as a researcher to lunch—not on that particular day, but rather the Rockefeller custom. "The dining room where I first met Dr. Avery was the greatest educational institution I have known anywhere," he wrote. "I came to the Institute not knowing a word about medicine. But every day in the dining room at lunch I became slowly sensitized....My suspicion is that if it had not been for the dining room at the Rockefeller I would not have been as rapidly successful in science."

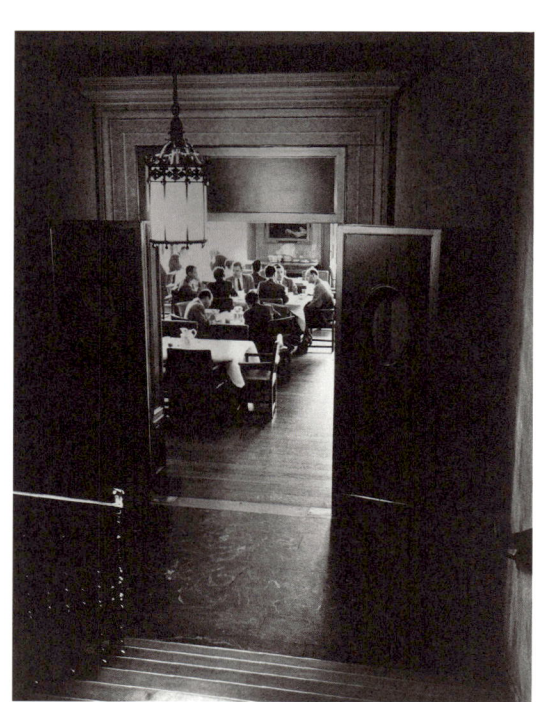

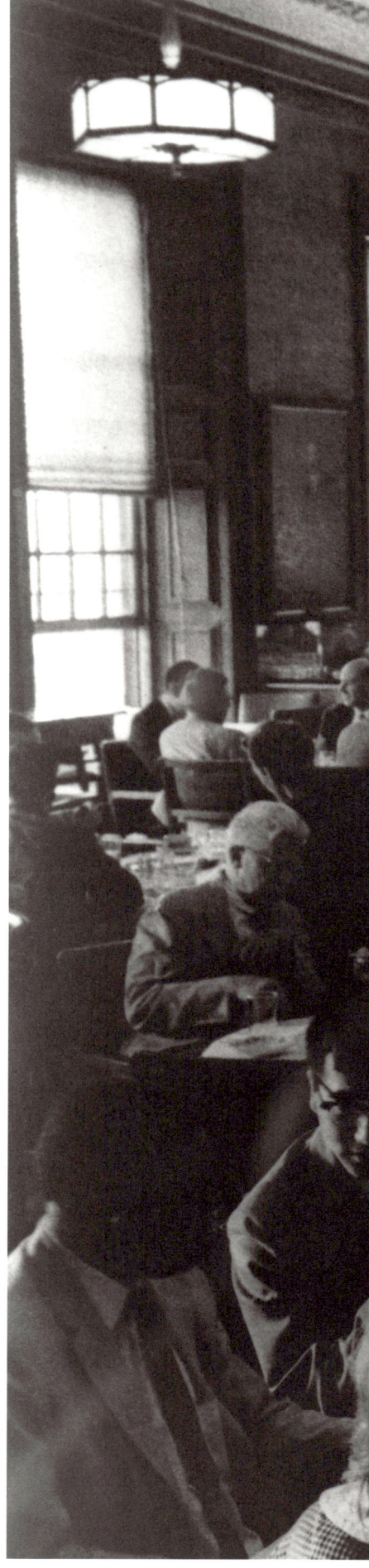

The dining room on the first floor of Welch Hall was an important gathering place for Rockefeller faculty.

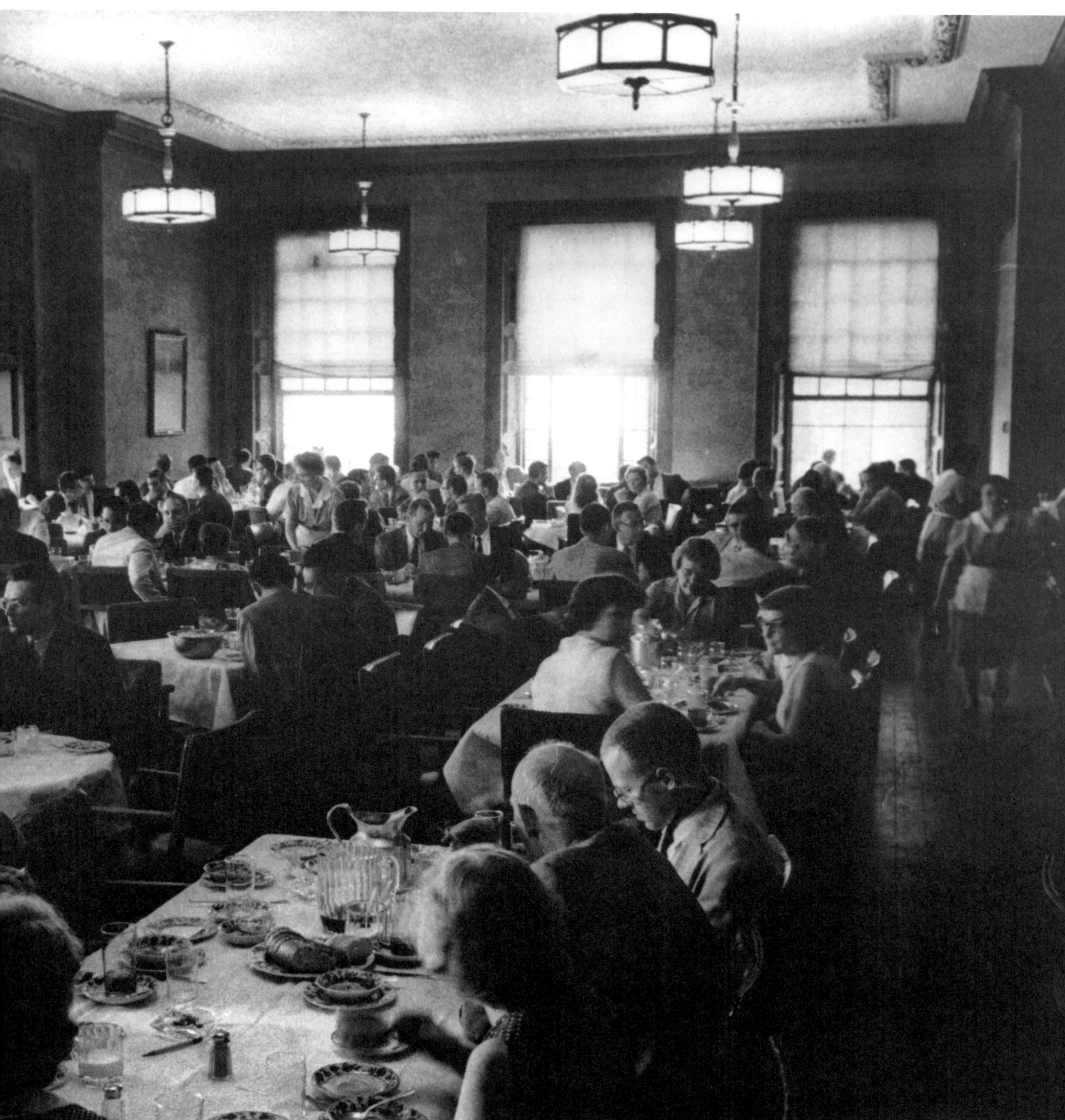

The Living Crystal

Wendell Stanley, a chemist working at The Rockefeller Institute's Princeton branch, became a scientific celebrity in the summer of 1935. He had purified a virus—a living infectious organism—in the form of needlelike crystals, which were inert, rigidly structured chemical formations. When Stanley dissolved the crystals in liquid and injected this into plants, the virus again produced disease. It also multiplied. The finding prompted debates over the essence of life. The Institute again made newspaper headlines. Had the border between living and nonliving been discovered?

Stanley experimented with the tobacco mosaic virus, a virus that infects plants, causing spots on their leaves. In the tradition of research at Rockefeller, he sought to understand its chemical nature. Stanley ground up the leaves of infected plants and extracted the virus from the plant juice using methods his Rockefeller colleague John Northrop had developed for crystallizing proteins. The highly concentrated substance indeed had the properties of a protein. Since conventional wisdom held that genes must be made of protein, Stanley's crystalline virus—seemingly purified as a protein and capable of reproducing itself—caused a sensation.

Following up on Stanley's work, other researchers soon found that his crystals were not pure protein. They contained a small amount of ribonucleic acid, or RNA. This RNA was responsible for the virus's reproductive powers. Nonetheless, Stanley's finding seemed to hold the key to understanding the chemistry of life. In 1946 Stanley, Northrop, and James B. Sumner shared the Nobel Prize in chemistry.

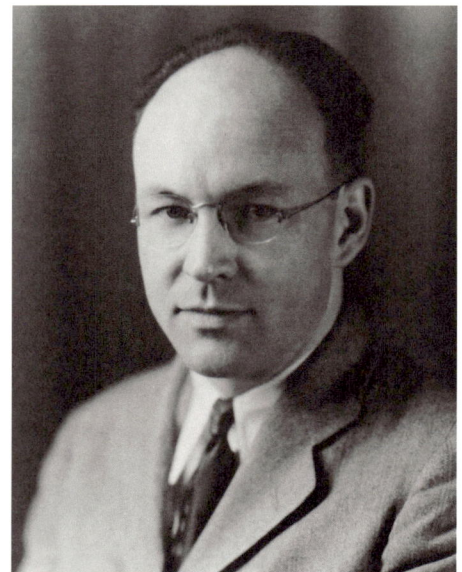

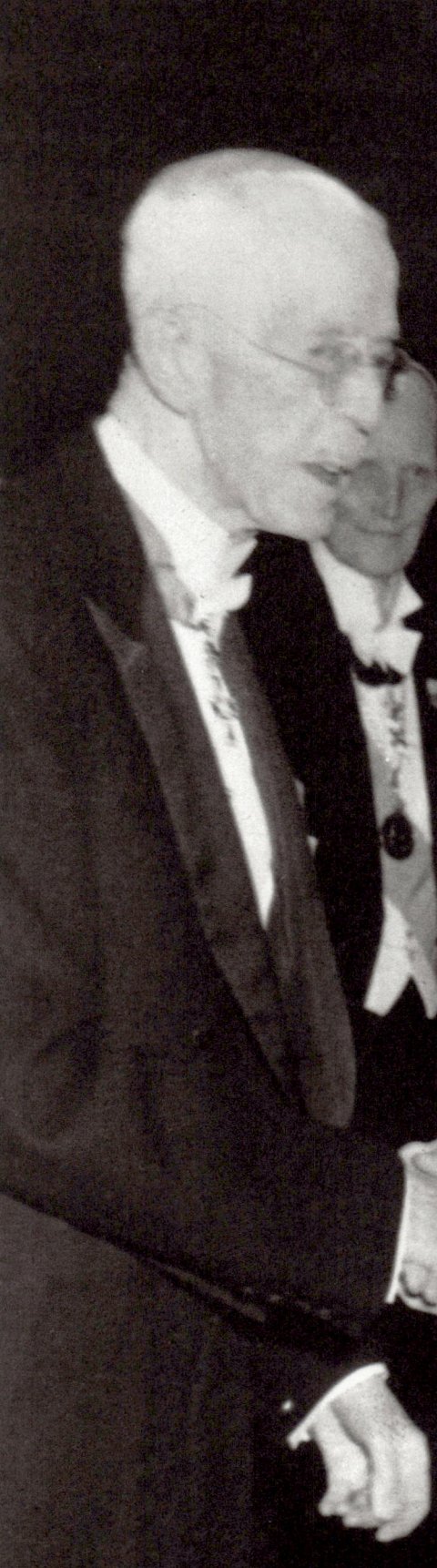

King Gustav of Sweden gives Nobel Prize diplomas to Wendell Stanley, John Northrop, and James Sumner in 1946.

When the Institute closed its Princeton branch Wendell Stanley moved to the University of California at Berkeley. There he founded the Virus Laboratory, bringing together leaders in the emerging discipline of virology in the 1950s and 1960s.

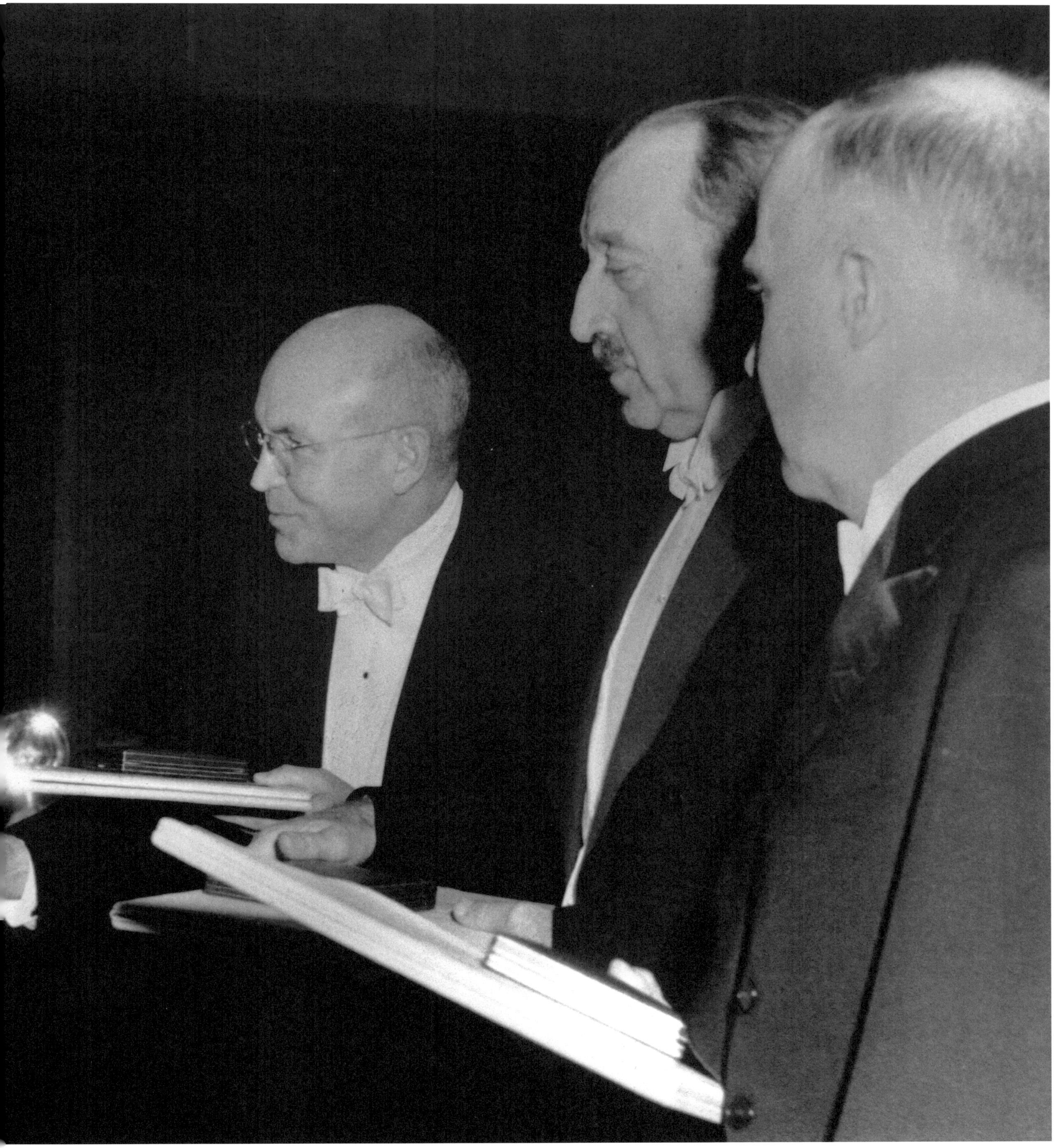

Karl Landsteiner

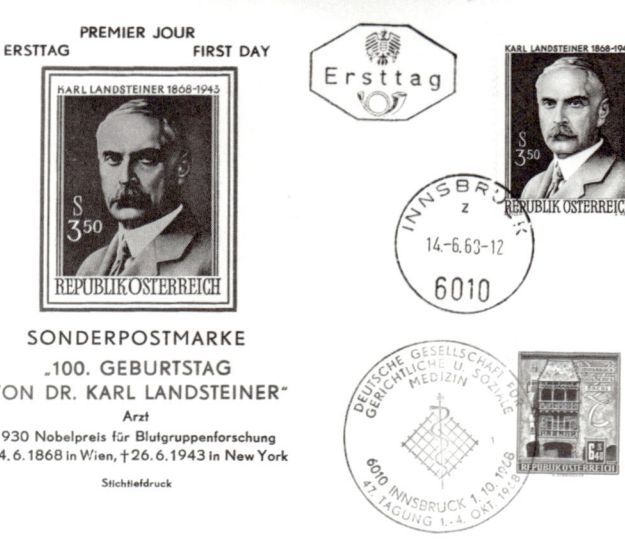

The Austrian government issued a commemorative postage stamp on June 14, 1968, the 100th anniversary of Karl Landsteiner's birth. Landsteiner inaugurated the study of immunology at Rockefeller, a research area that continues to thrive today.

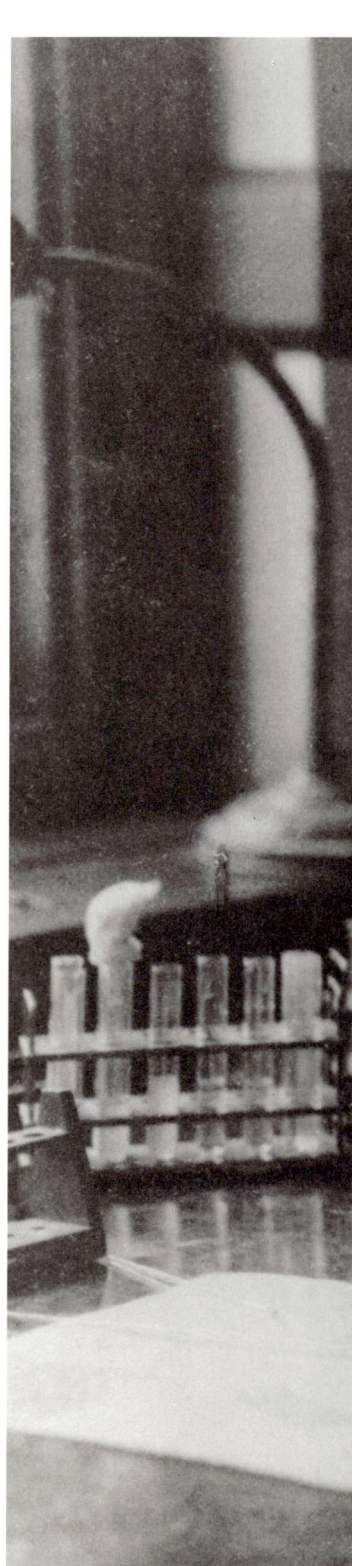

Karl Landsteiner, born and educated in Vienna, had been studying the chemistry of immunological reactions for nearly 30 years by the time he was appointed to The Rockefeller Institute in 1922. In 1900 he classified human blood into four groups, based on immunological reactions. This discovery of blood types made transfusions safe, and for this work Landsteiner was awarded a Nobel Prize in 1930.

In Vienna, Landsteiner had conducted his prodigious research under difficult conditions; he also taught medical students and served as chief pathologist at a large hospital. In the aftermath of World War I, however, scientific work became impossible and Landsteiner lost much of his personal property.

Seeing no future in Austria, Landsteiner accepted an appointment at a small Roman Catholic hospital in The Hague, where he did routine postmortems, and tissue, blood, urine, and Wassermann tests. One of Landsteiner's friends wrote to Simon Flexner describing the scientist's frustration: "He has to do all this with the assistance of a single Roman Catholic nurse who is at the same time the organist of the hospital church, and in only one room. Moreover, the nurse pours out coffee for doctors and assistants, sometimes leaves the laboratory to go and pray in the church, etc."

In 1921 the Board of Directors of The Rockefeller Institute invited Landsteiner to visit for a conference. Later that year they appointed him a Member of the Institute. He was 54 years old when given this first opportunity in his career to pursue research full-time, and he threw himself into his work with an intensity that impressed all who knew him.

At Rockefeller, Landsteiner devoted much of his research to the chemical analysis of immune reactions. He synthesized artificial antigens, which he called haptens, and showed that antibodies could be directed toward molecules of known chemical structure, a founding principle of immunochemistry. He also detailed many of the ways in which antibody specificity depends on chemical structure. Landsteiner's interest in the mechanisms of allergic reaction led him to discover the Rh factor in blood—the antigen that can make a pregnant woman's body reject her fetus.

Landsteiner's personal qualities—he was modest, diligent, exacting, and intolerant of idleness—were as legendary as his achievements in the laboratory. Profoundly self-critical, he did not at first tell his family when newspapers announced his Nobel Prize for fear they would be disappointed if the news were not true.

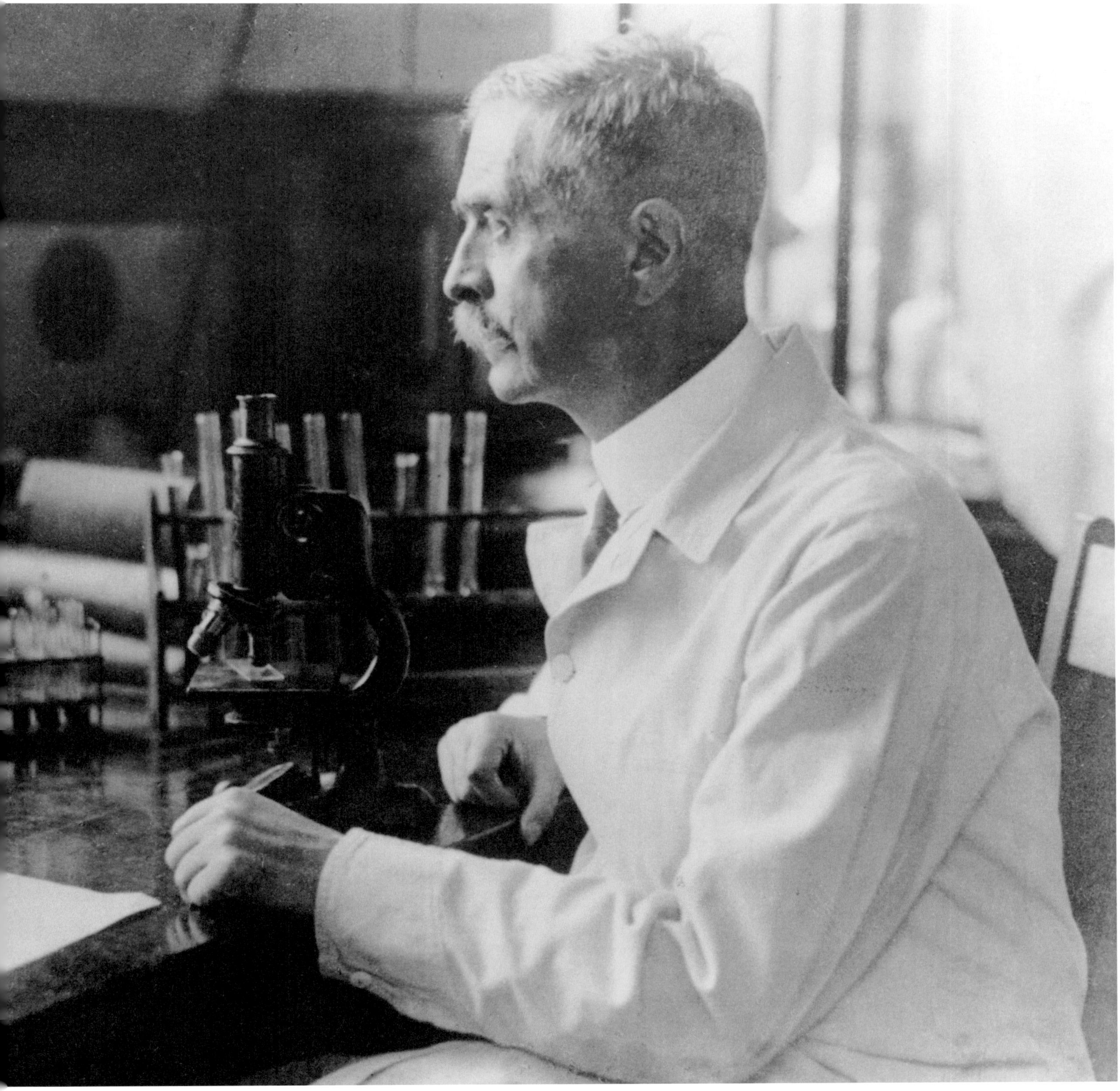

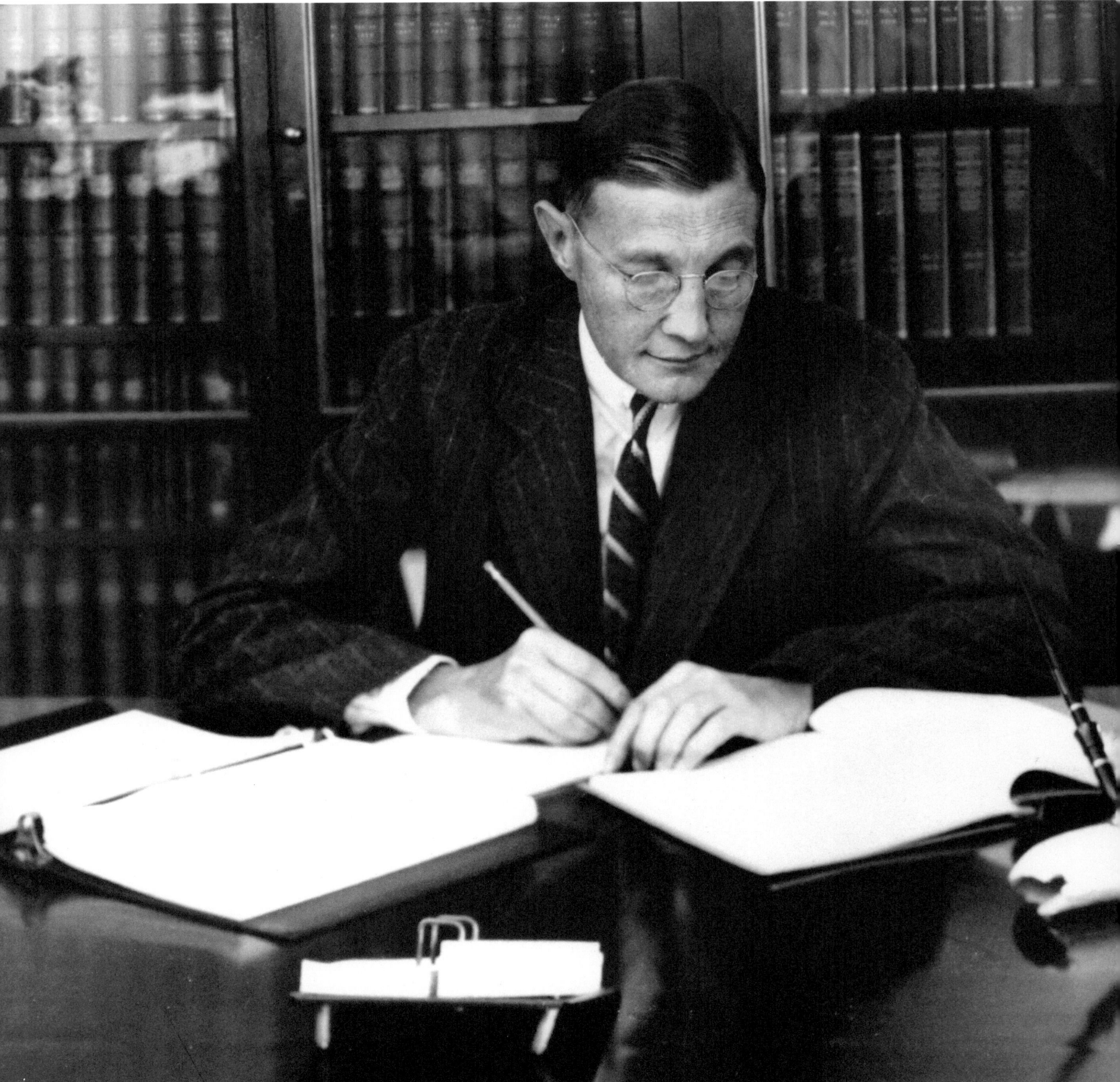

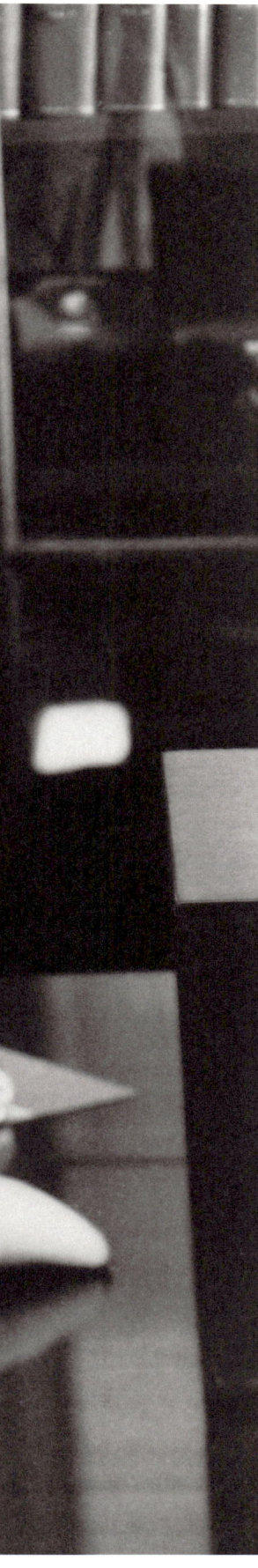

Herbert Gasser

Herbert Spencer Gasser became the second director of The Rockefeller Institute in 1935. Since 1931 he had been a professor of physiology at Cornell University Medical College. As a neighbor of The Rockefeller Institute staff and a colleague of the president of Rockefeller's Board of Scientific Directors, Gasser was well known at the Institute. He had spent most of his earlier career at Washington University in St. Louis, where he developed electrophysiological techniques for studying nerves. For these studies into the nature of nerve conduction, carried out with Joseph Erlanger, Gasser and Erlanger were awarded a Nobel Prize in 1944.

As director, Gasser strengthened and expanded research in the basic biological sciences at the Institute. Remarkable advances in understanding infectious disease had been made under Flexner; now Gasser shifted the focus of attention to understanding fundamental life processes at the level of the cell. He broadened the areas of research at the Institute, brought in the first biophysicists, supported work in physical chemistry, and launched studies into the structure and function of the nervous system.

Gasser took a keen interest in the research of every investigator, subjecting their annual reports to the Board of Scientific Directors to unprecedented scrutiny. According to an often-told anecdote, he once queried biochemists Stanford Moore and William Stein about a small peak on a chart they had submitted. Moore and Stein had initially passed over this bit of data; when they followed it up, they were able to isolate a new compound.

As an administrator, Gasser continued Flexner's practice of allowing researchers to work in freedom. "About new knowledge two points are clear," he wrote. "It cannot be forecast; and it cannot be achieved through administrative action. All that can be done is to create optimal conditions for its production." In subtle ways, however, he made changes to the infrastructure of the Institute. For example, under Flexner, when a member of the Institute retired or died the laboratory was disbanded and its staff left the Institute. Gasser, in contrast, often encouraged talented scientific staff to stay at the Institute in such cases, and occasionally allowed a senior scientist to take over as head of the laboratory.

Herbert Gasser in his Founder's Hall office.

Science and War

During the First World War the Institute had been commissioned as an Army post and this involvement had disrupted normal research activities. In 1940 and 1941 it became clear that the United States was headed toward involvement in another conflict and Thomas Rivers, the director of the Rockefeller Hospital, made plans then to integrate the coming war effort into the ongoing work of the Institute. He felt this would prevent a radical shift in the Institute's research priorities.

The Navy was concerned with potential epidemics of pneumonia and scarlet fever. These diseases already were under study at the Hospital, so the Institute made a dollar-a-year contract with the Brooklyn Naval Hospital to receive Navy patients. Rivers accepted a Commander's position in the Navy Medical Reserve Corps and encouraged his staff to join the Corps. The Naval Research Unit at the Hospital of The Rockefeller Institute began receiving military patients in 1942 and operated through June 1946. Rivers also headed a unit based in Guam in 1944 and 1945 to investigate the danger of tropical diseases to Allied forces.

Outbreaks of rheumatic fever and scarlet fever in military barracks provided an opportunity for research on how these diseases are transmitted. At Rockefeller, Rebecca Lancefield was well known for her work on classifying the streptococcal bacteria, associating bacterial types with specific diseases. During the war, Lancefield worked with the Naval Medical Center, the Army's Board for Investigation of Epidemic Diseases, and others to type bacterial cultures isolated from patients in military hospitals. The evidence from the thousands of cultures that she typed informed later studies on streptococcal epidemiology and the mechanism by which rheumatic fever develops after a streptococcal infection with scarlet fever. The data also led to a practical immediate recommendation for smaller barracks to reduce the chance of infectious outbreaks.

Among wartime scientific assignments at Rockefeller, perhaps the most adventurous fell to Richard Shope, who came under fire in 1945 while searching for malaria-carrying mosquitoes and other pathogenic organisms in Okinawa. Fear of biological warfare prompted another project. In 1942, the Secretary of War had directed Shope to produce a vaccine against the virus that causes rinderpest, a disease of cattle. Shope worked on the vaccine in secret for 19 months in a laboratory on an island in the St. Lawrence River near Quebec City.

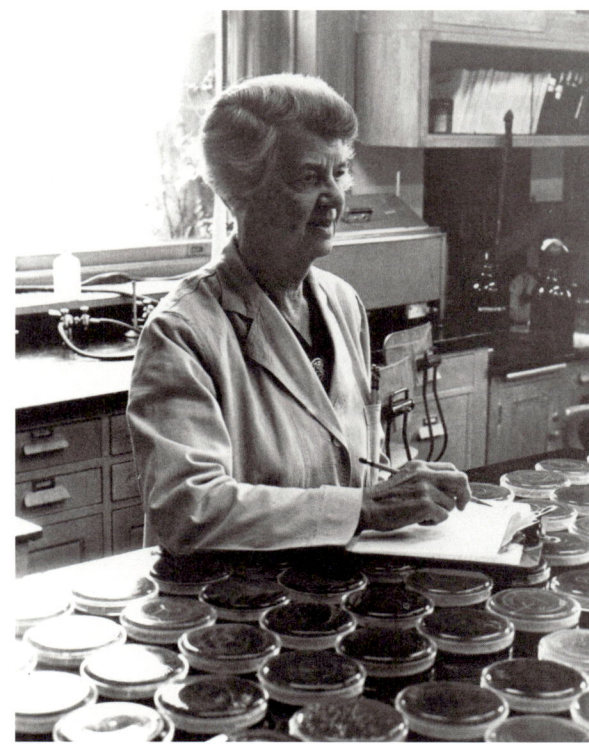

Rebecca Lancefield joined the Institute in 1918 and became a world-renowned authority on the streptococcal bacteria, which cause rheumatic fever, scarlet fever, and other diseases.

U.S. Naval Medical Research Unit No. 2 in Guam, where Rockefeller's Thomas Rivers and others investigated infectious diseases. Left to right: Steve Holt, Horace L. Hodes, Thomas Rivers, and Basil O'Connor, chairman of the American Red Cross. (1945)

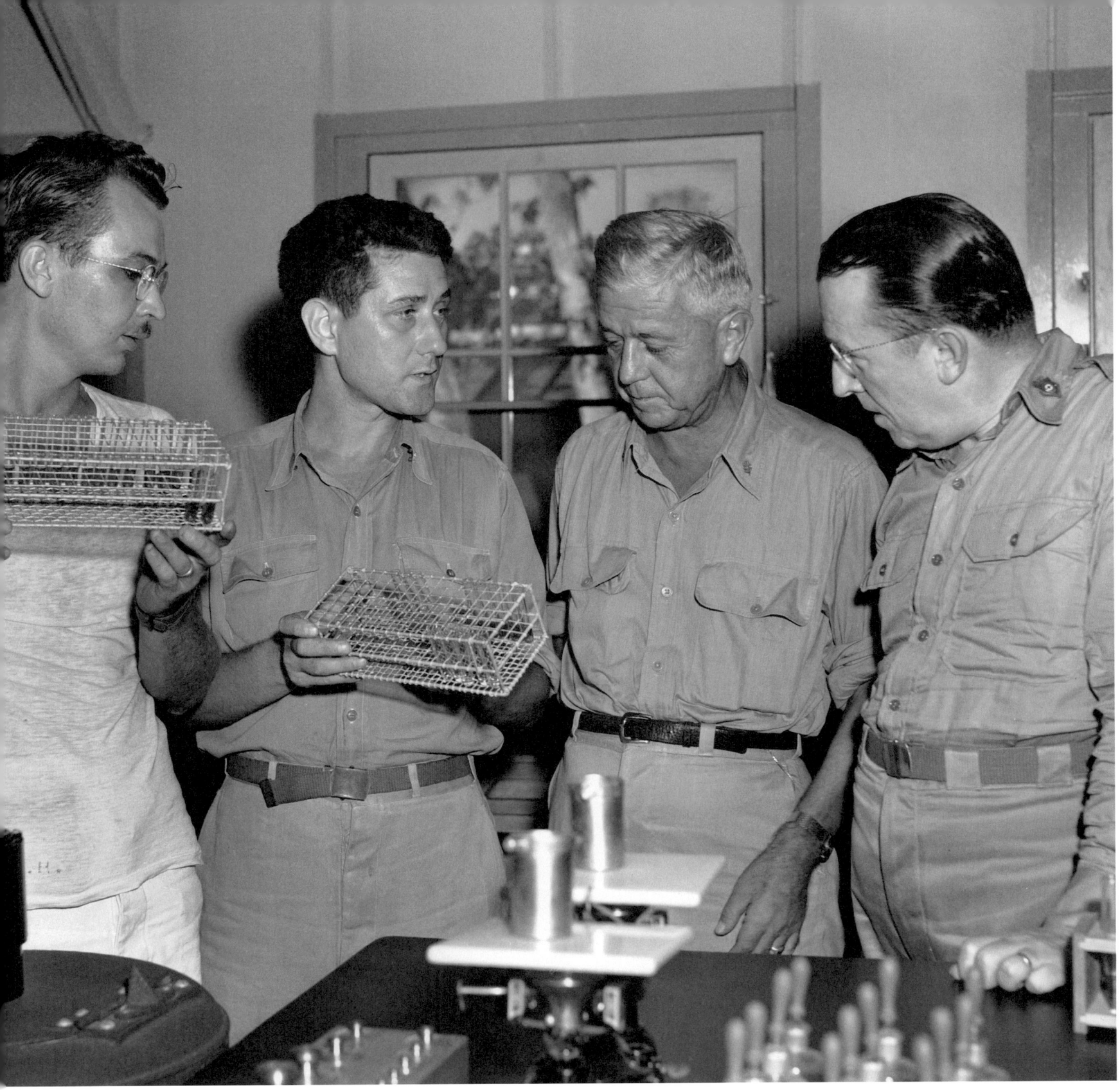

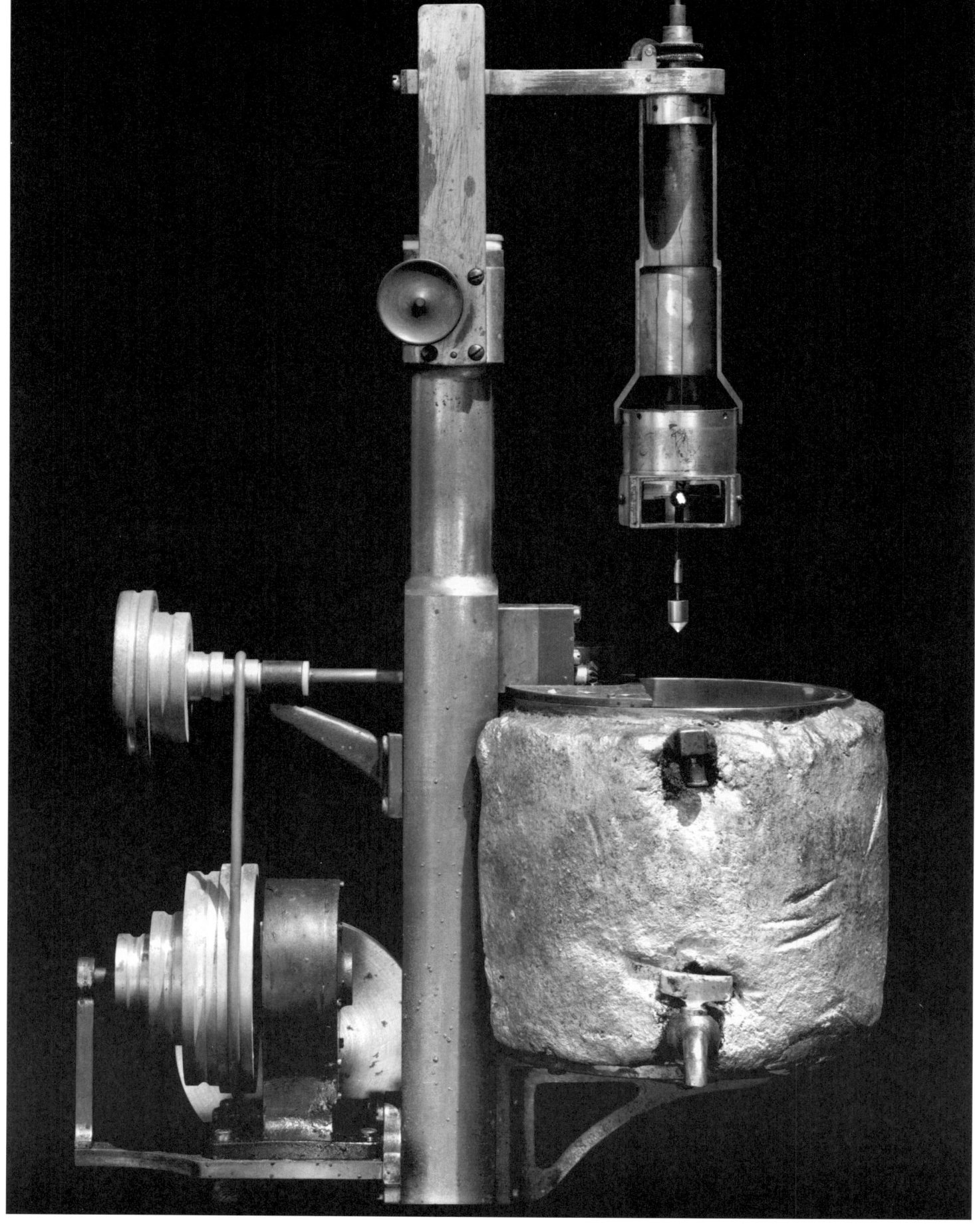

Tools for Discovery

Rotating disk viscometer, used in the 1920s in the laboratory of Alexis Carrel to gauge the viscosity of liquids.

Glassblower Wolfgang Papperitz at work around 1965. With commercial glassware readily available and little demand for unique pieces, the glassblower's shop closed in 2000.

Many scientific advances at Rockefeller have gone hand in hand with the development of new instruments. Scientists have invented their own devices to measure nerve impulses or separate and purify chemical compounds. Today instruments are usually mass-produced by commercial manufacturers. But for much of the century that was not the case, and Rockefeller was unique in keeping skilled craftsmen on staff in the instrument, electronics, and glassblower's shops. Work in these shops ranged from routine repairs on existing instruments to producing one-of-a-kind centrifuges and other inventions designed to meet specific laboratory needs.

Early in the Institute's history, much research depended on uniquely designed glass flasks and tubing. The pump developed by Alexis Carrel and pioneering aviator Charles Lindbergh for perfusing organs with oxygenated blood is one example. Lindbergh, a skilled engineer as well as a pilot, worked as a volunteer in Carrel's laboratory in the early 1930s designing the pump and working with the Institute's glassblower and instrument shop to create it. This complex apparatus was a step toward making organ transplants possible.

In the 1950s Rockefeller's instrument makers developed a new version of a device called a microtome. This instrument slices specimens into thin sections so that researchers can look at them with a microscope. The new microtome was adapted to the needs of viewing cells with an electron microscope. The ability to create appropriate specimens was essential to cell biology as it developed at Rockefeller, for it enabled scientists to see cellular organelles clearly.

In recent decades, scientific practice has come to rely on computers as much as on mechanical instruments. Even here the University remains a center for invention, with faculty and technical staff developing prototype programs for gene mapping and comparing the genomes of different organisms.

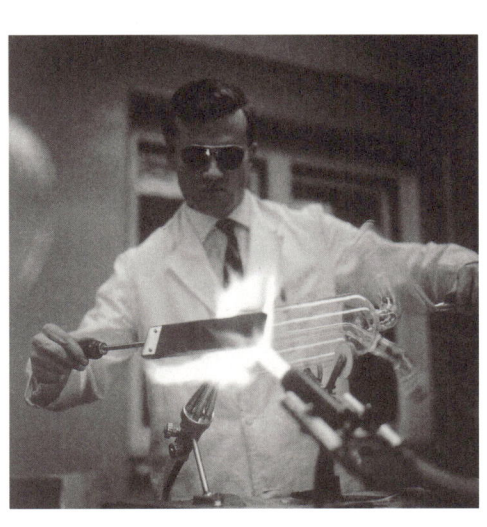
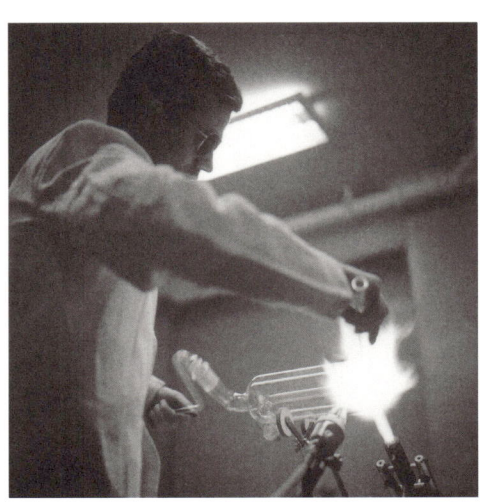
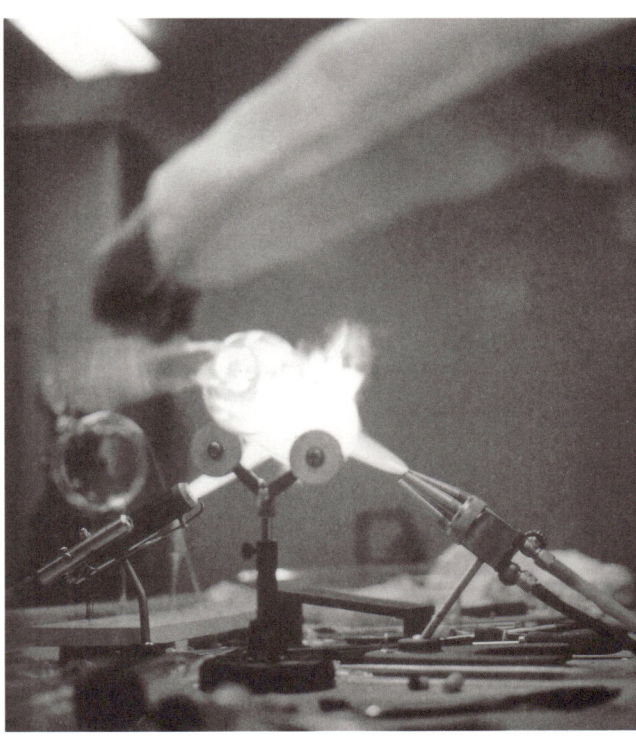

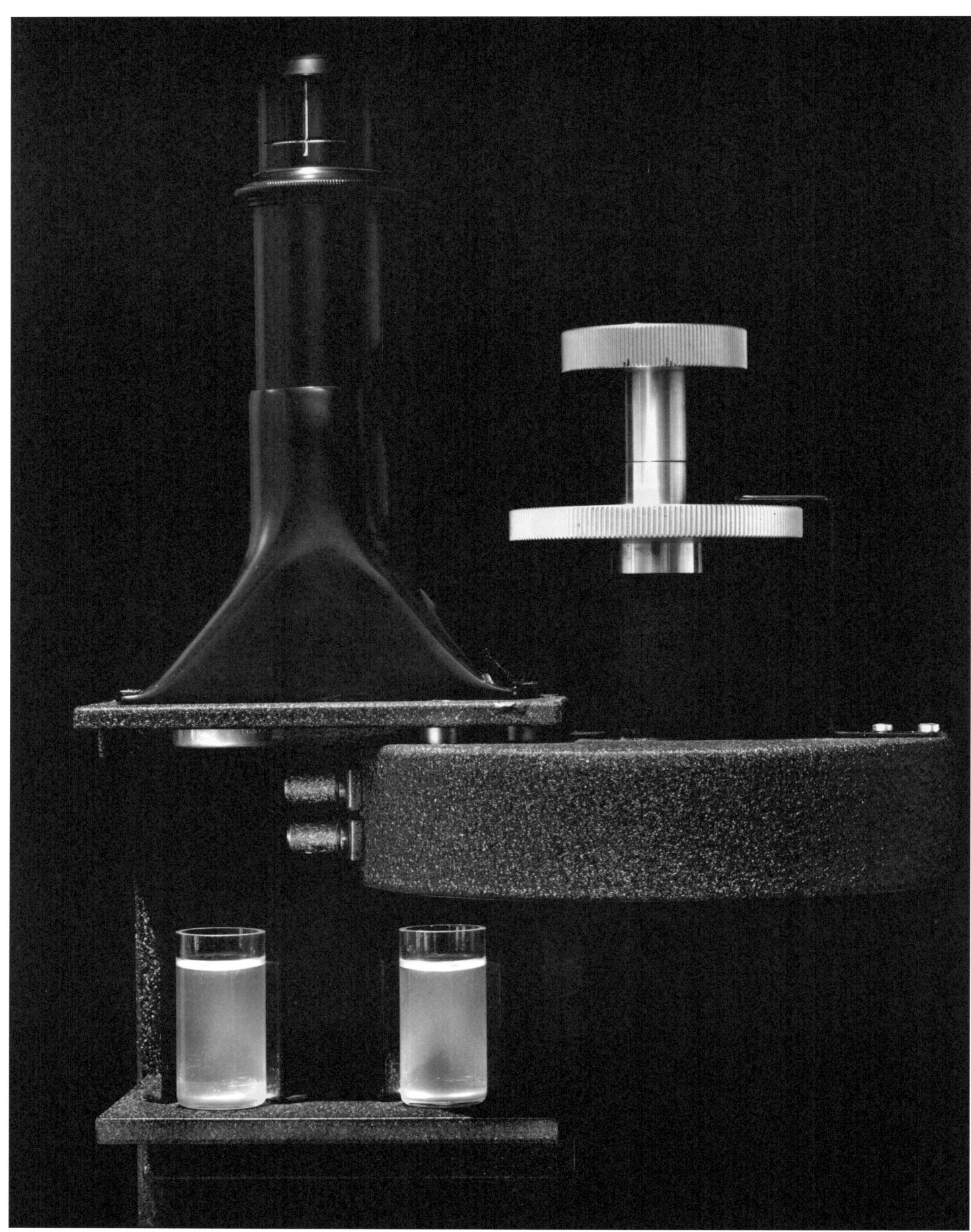

Photometer, used by Donald Van Slyke for determining the plasma volume of blood samples.

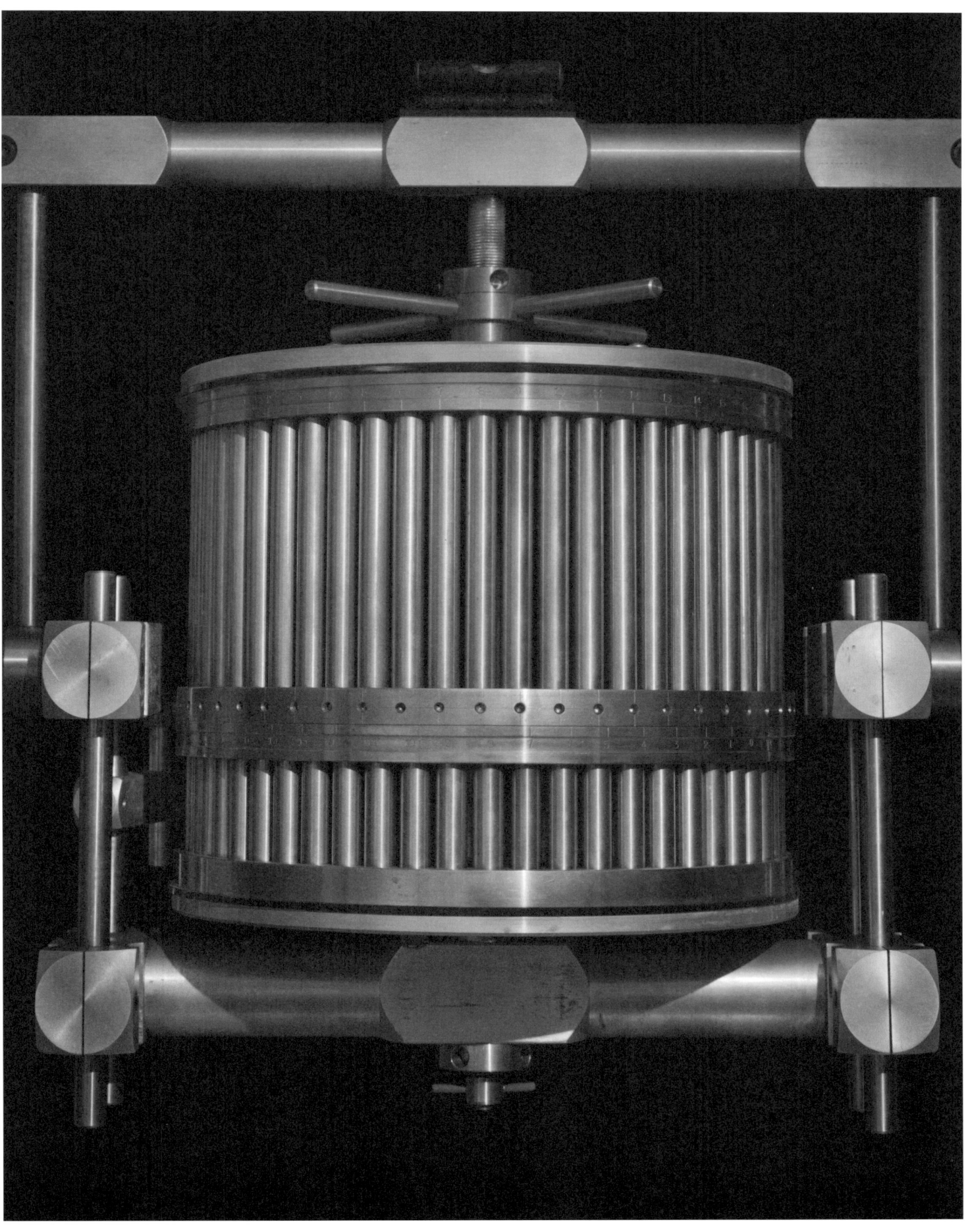
Countercurrent distribution apparatus for separating complex chemical mixtures, developed in the early 1940s by Lyman Craig.

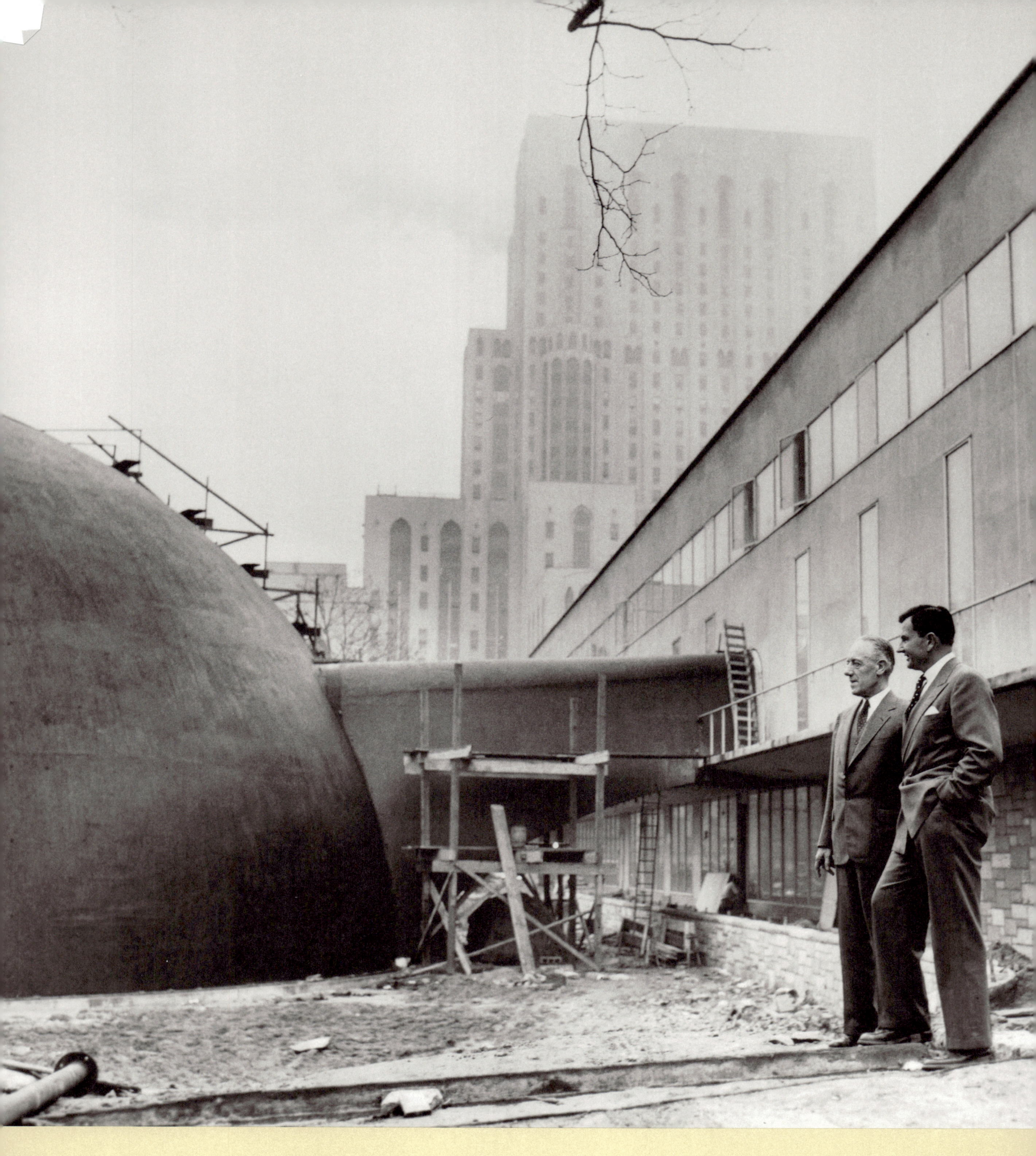

GROWTH

Part 3: From Institute to University

In the late 1940s, at a high point in its scientific achievements, The Rockefeller Institute for Medical Research suffered a form of identity crisis. The Institute was no longer unique. In the 50 years since its conception, scientific research had grown from a cottage industry into the acknowledged responsibility of every large university. Dozens of new hospitals had been organized around the paradigm of clinical research set forth at the Rockefeller Hospital. The United States government had begun funding science on an unprecedented level, and plans for vastly expanding the National Institutes of Health were under way. "No longer does it hold that medical research is what is done by a few valiant spirits as best they can without support, and in ill-equipped laboratories," wrote Herbert Gasser, the Institute's director. "Medical research has acquired a sweep and momentum."

The Institute's own success contributed to its crisis—researchers trained at Rockefeller became leaders at new institutions. During the Institute's first half century, 650 men and women had served on the research staff in ranks below that of Member. By 1953, 200 of them held full professorships or equivalent positions in research institutes, industry, and public service in 31 states and 16 countries. The Rockefeller Institute for Medical Research had fulfilled its founding goals to expand medical knowledge, set high research standards for others to follow, train scientists, and foster widespread respect for science and the scientific method. It was now time to examine its future goals.

Detlev Bronk (left) and David Rockefeller survey the construction of Caspary Hall and Auditorium.

In 1946 John D. Rockefeller Jr., who was president of the Board of Trustees, initiated a period of self-reflection for the Institute by asking director Herbert Gasser for a report on its future policy. In 1950 Rockefeller Jr. stepped down as president of the board, and his son David succeeded him. In the following years David Rockefeller would guide the trustees through a thorough evaluation of the Institute's past and strategic planning for its future. Over the next decade, new leaders would bring students to Rockefeller, renovate the campus, and begin new traditions while maintaining the integrity of the institution's commitments to basic research and scientific excellence.

Most immediately, however, financial and scientific considerations convinced the trustees to close the Institute's branch in Princeton. The facilities there duplicated some of those in New York, which was costly, especially since economic depression and war in the 1930s and 1940s had strained the Institute's financial resources. Members of the Board of Scientific Directors maintained that most investigations of animal diseases had turned toward the laboratory study of viruses and parasites and no longer required rural facilities for keeping swine or sheep. By the time the Princeton laboratories closed in 1950, half the staff had resigned. The remainder relocated to the Institute's New York campus.

On the question of how the Institute should maintain its vitality, the trustees consulted the leading scientific administrators and educators of the day—Warren Weaver at the Rockefeller Foundation, Robert Oppenheimer at the Institute for Advanced Study, James Shannon at the new National Heart Institute, and Vannevar Bush at the Carnegie Institution, among dozens of others. A deliberate effort was made to consider all options seriously, and their advice was wide ranging. Some suggested that, since Rockefeller's founding mission had been achieved, the Institute should close its doors and put its endowment toward establishing research professorships at various universities. Others raised the issue of teaching. Scientists at Rockefeller and elsewhere had long debated whether the influx of fresh ideas from students was a fair exchange for the time away from research that was required to instruct them. Those who felt that teaching should be combined with research proposed that the Institute relinquish its independent status and affiliate with a university. Closing the Hospital was also suggested, on the premise that publicly funded institutions could pick up where Rockefeller left off. Other advisors supported concentrating efforts on basic biological science rather than medical research broadly construed. Faculty members consulted on the Institute's future

Vision Research

Since the 1950s Rockefeller has been home to remarkable research on the complex interactions between eye and brain that result in perhaps the most acute of human senses—vision. H. Keffer Hartline continued research here that would win him a 1967 Nobel Prize, examining the light receptors and electrophysiology of the eye of the horseshoe crab. Floyd Ratliff and Bruce Knight came to Rockefeller to join Hartline's laboratory. Neurobiological research continues today in the laboratories of Knight and Rockefeller president emeritus and professor Torsten Wiesel, winner of a 1981 Nobel Prize for studies of how visual information is transmitted from the retina to the brain.

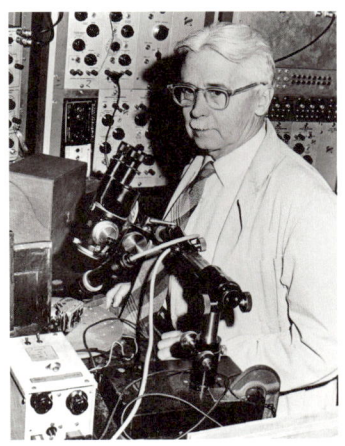

H. Keffer Hartline in 1965.

voiced hope for preserving its open structure, to which they attributed the Institute's productivity, and for continuing the support of individuals pursuing long-term projects.

During this process Herbert Gasser decided to retire as director of the Institute and the subcommittee of the trustees that was evaluating the recommendations also began searching for a new director. The chairman of the subcommittee was Detlev W. Bronk, known for his talents both as a scientist and as an administrator. At the time he was a member of Rockefeller's Board of Scientific Directors, president of Johns Hopkins University, and president of the National Academy of Sciences. After all options had been laid out, Bronk persuaded the committee that the Institute should become a graduate university, bringing young scientists to campus and formalizing a long tradition of postgraduate education in its laboratories. In addition, Bronk recommended dropping the words "for Medical Research" from the Institute's title, strengthening support for basic research in the life sciences, and initiating research in areas not traditionally represented at the Institute.

In 1953 the trustees voted to incorporate the Institute as a graduate university empowered to grant the degree of doctor of philosophy. Bronk was appointed to the new title of president. "As time went on it became clear that the person who had the sharpest vision of where the Institute ought to be going was Dr. Bronk himself," recalls David Rockefeller. "He had the most and the best ideas."

At the same time, the Board of Trustees merged with the Board of Scientific Directors to form a single Board of Trustees with David Rockefeller as chairman. The Institute received its new charter as a degree-granting organization in 1954, and faculty who had been titled "Members of the Institute" became "Professors." In 1965 the Institute's name was changed to The Rockefeller University.

The first class of ten graduate students came to Rockefeller in 1955. They entered a program that was unlike any other curriculum of advanced training in the sciences, with few formal courses and no examinations. What Rockefeller offered was an opportunity for students to join a community of scholars as junior colleagues, pursuing independent research, and learning through daily mentoring in the laboratory. The University charged no tuition and provided a stipend for living expenses. To find young scientists capable of self-directed study, Bronk asked college presidents and heads of science departments around the country to recommend their best graduates. Bronk himself interviewed most prospective Rockefeller students during his presidency.

Bronk's idea for a graduate university developed during the years when he was simultaneously discussing academic policy with the faculty of Johns Hopkins and chairing the committee that was planning the future of Rockefeller. Bronk admired the philosophy of Johns Hopkins' founding president Daniel Coit Gilman, who established it in 1876 as the first research university in the United States based on the German tradition. Gilman emphasized research and scholarship as the core activities of a modern university, and while he led Hopkins, Bronk extended Gilman's ideas by de-emphasizing distinctions between undergraduate and graduate education to promote both research and interdisciplinary study.

He refined these ideas in his plan to make Rockefeller a graduate university. Higher education in the sciences requires specialization, but Bronk wanted Rockefeller graduates to leave with a wide scientific and cultural outlook, and broad knowledge outside their areas of expertise. The city of New York was an ideal location to try out his ideas because it readily provided students with opportunities to appreciate the arts—indeed, student stipends allowed for concert and theater tickets. Bronk also invited musicians, writers, and others to weekly dinners with students and faculty as a way of making up for the lack of a faculty in the humanities.

The first Ph.D. degrees from Rockefeller were conferred in 1959. At Convocation in June of that year Bronk set in place a tradition that celebrates Rockefeller's unique graduate program. "An occasion such as this is fraught with temptation to speak of many things regarding science and education and the objectives of ourselves and our Institute and our nation," Bronk said. "But I have vowed that our Commencement should be for those whom we would honor rather than for a speaker to the public which seldom listens." With that he turned the program over to the faculty mentors of the new graduates, who presented the achievements of each student individually.

The completion of several new buildings on the campus provided another reason for celebration in the spring of 1959. Creating an environment that would nurture scientific creativity was as important to Bronk's vision for Rockefeller as bringing in students. When Bronk arrived in 1953, Rockefeller's physical plant was decades old and lacked many of the amenities of university life. The Welch Hall dining room provided a meeting place for faculty at lunch time, and its role in the Institute's intellectual life was legendary. But there was no lecture hall, no place for the informal social gatherings so important to academic exchange, and no housing for the new students. Laboratory space was at a premium. Bronk went further than remedying these shortcomings; he embarked on a building program that is his most visible legacy to the University.

Cell Biology

Since researchers here first focused the electron microscope on the interiors of cells in the 1940s, Rockefeller has been a leader in the field of cell biology, with work twice recognized by Nobel Prizes. In the 1950s and 1960s Rockefeller scientists advanced the understanding of the internal structures of cells and their biochemical functions. These achievements and the continuing work of the next generations of cell biologists have answered fundamental questions of biology with implications for treating human disease.

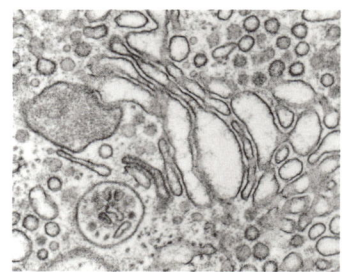

This electron micrograph of a rat pancreas cell shows the Golgi complex. The image is from the laboratory of George Palade.

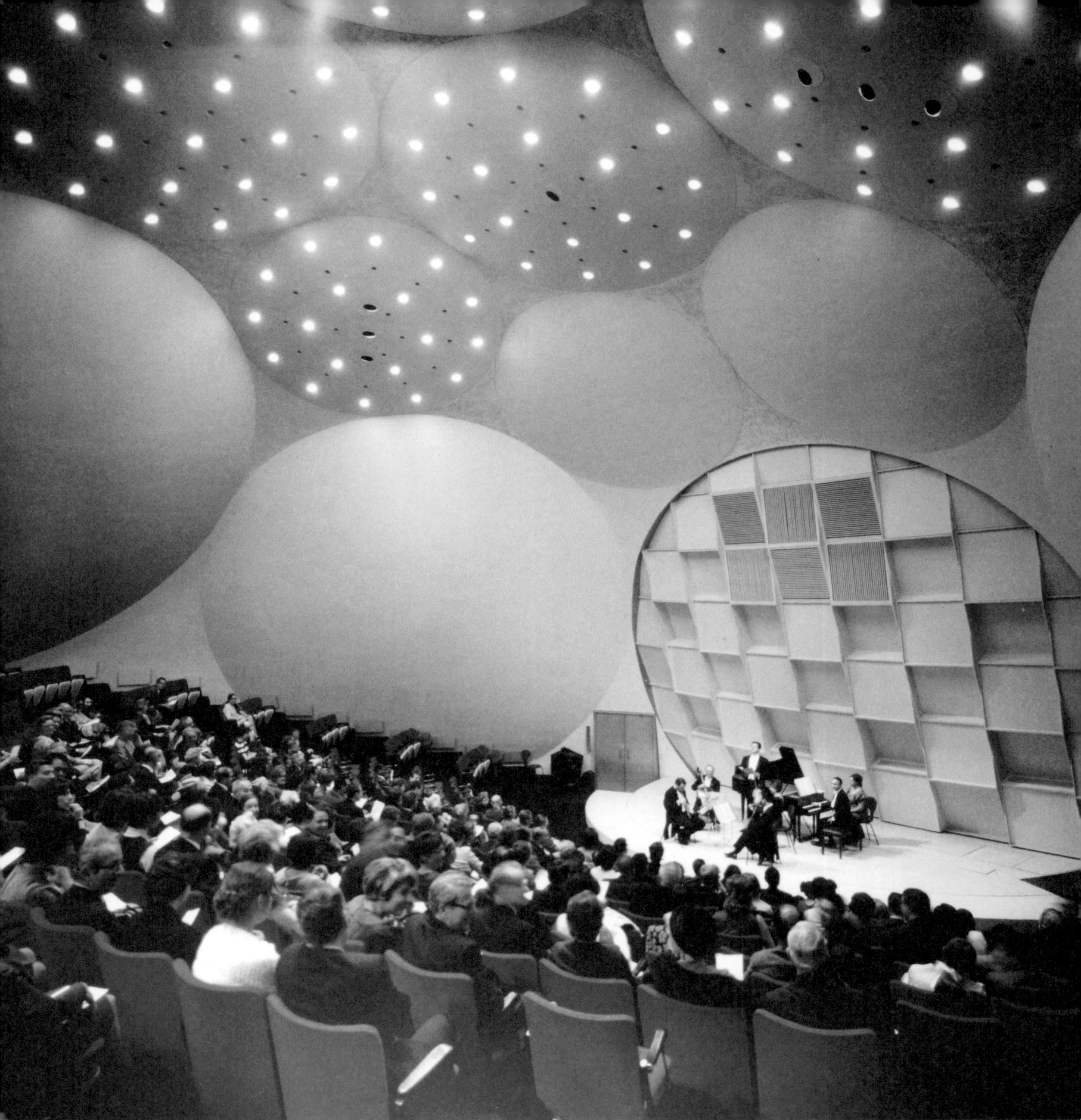

With the construction of Caspary Auditorium, Bronk created a place on campus for concerts and lectures.

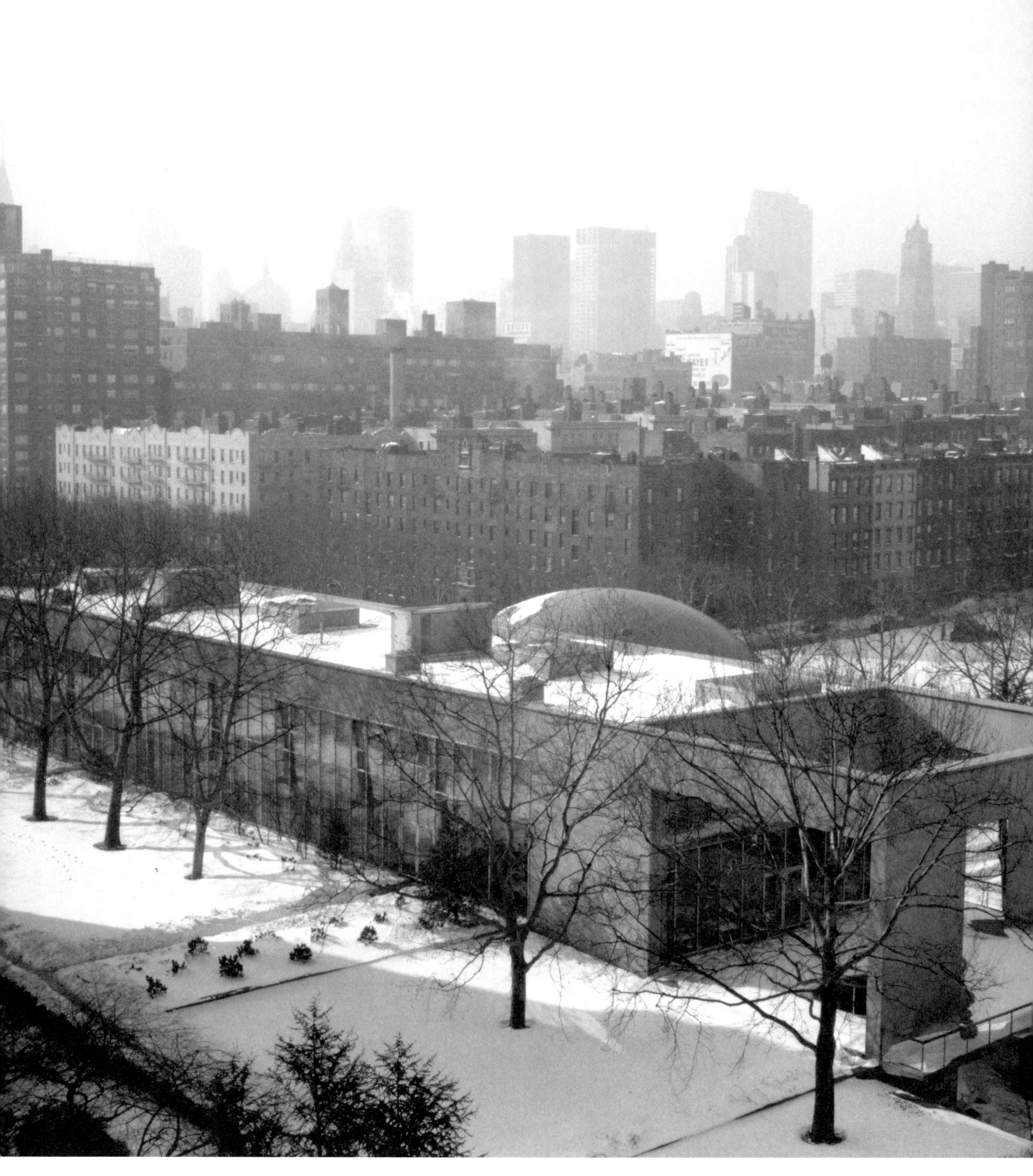

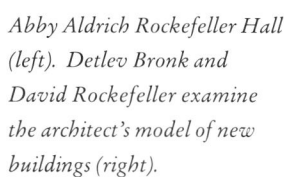

Abby Aldrich Rockefeller Hall (left). Detlev Bronk and David Rockefeller examine the architect's model of new buildings (right).

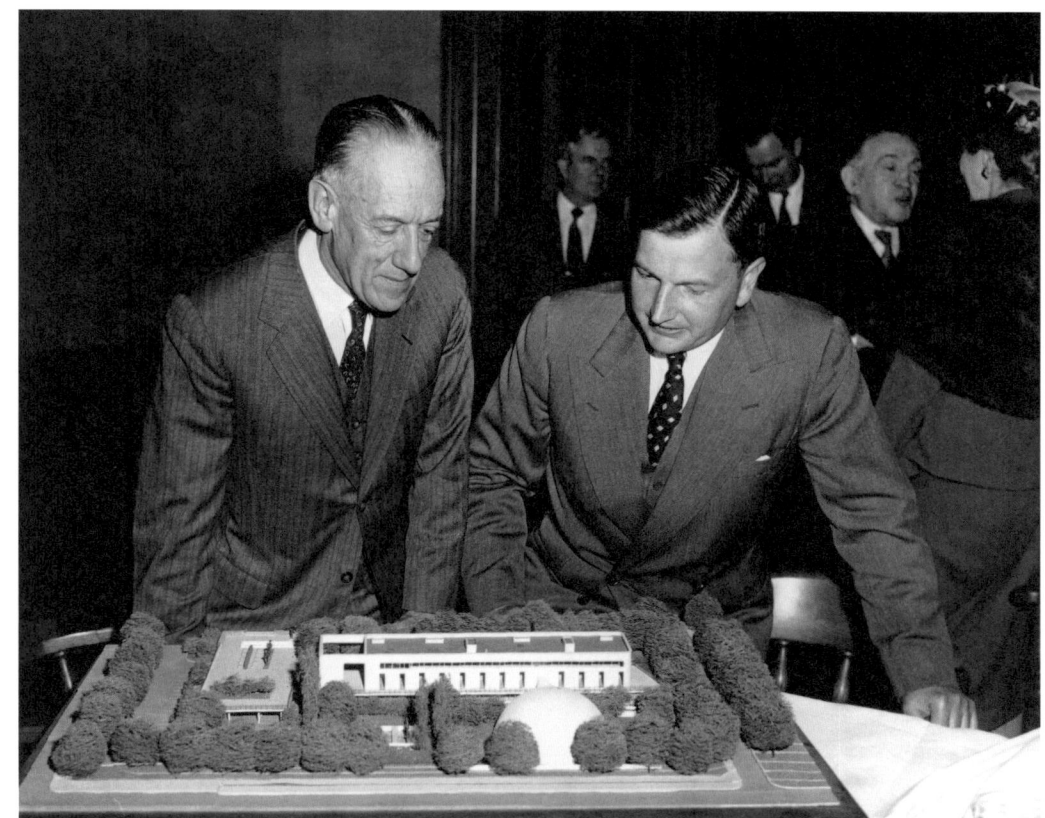

As architect, Bronk hired Wallace Harrison, who was already well known for designing the United Nations headquarters and much of Rockefeller Center. Harrison shared Bronk's commitment to creating an environment that would stimulate intellectual life. At the dedication of the buildings Harrison remarked, "This home for scientists… will always be an example of how the arts may aid the sciences by providing an atmosphere for easier and more effective communication of ideas between friends and fellow students." In the late 1950s the firm of Harrison and Abramovitz designed Abby Aldrich Rockefeller Hall, which has meeting areas, guest rooms for visitors, and a faculty and students club. They also designed Caspary Hall, Caspary Auditorium, the President's House, the Graduate Students Residence Hall, the Sophie Fricke Residence Hall, and Bronk Laboratory, which was at first called South Laboratory.

The Institute also acquired a collection of paintings, mainly postwar works by American abstract expressionists that were hung in Abby Aldrich Rockefeller Hall. Abby Aldrich Rockefeller was a founder of New York's Museum of Modern Art and Alfred Barr, then director of the museum, selected the works with his assistant Dorothy Miller. It seemed fitting to display the work of contemporary artists in the building dedicated to the memory of Abby Aldrich Rockefeller. Furthermore, the building celebrated the common creative impulses of science and art, gathering explorers of scientific knowledge in the midst of art that was on the frontier of aesthetic expression.

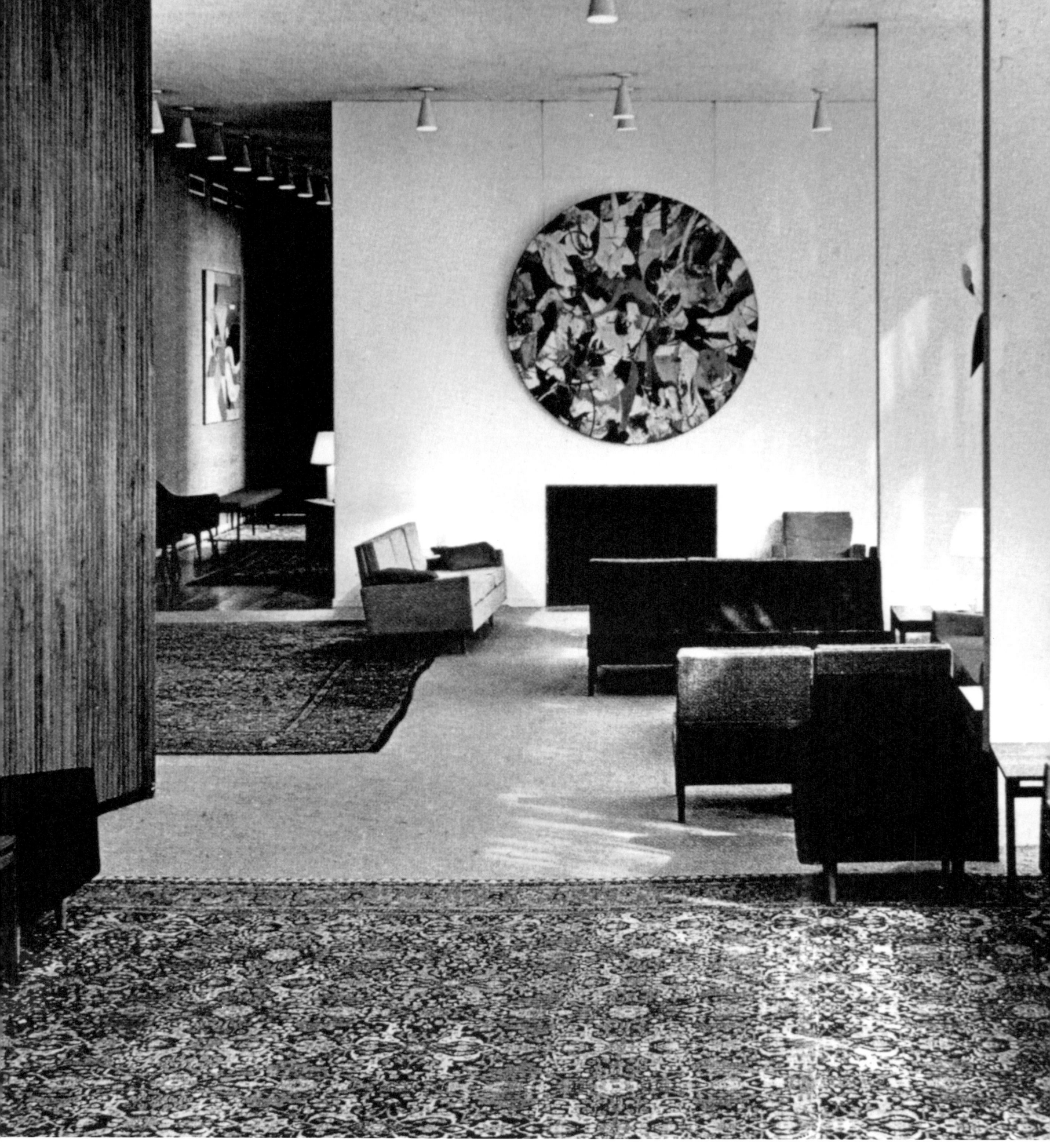

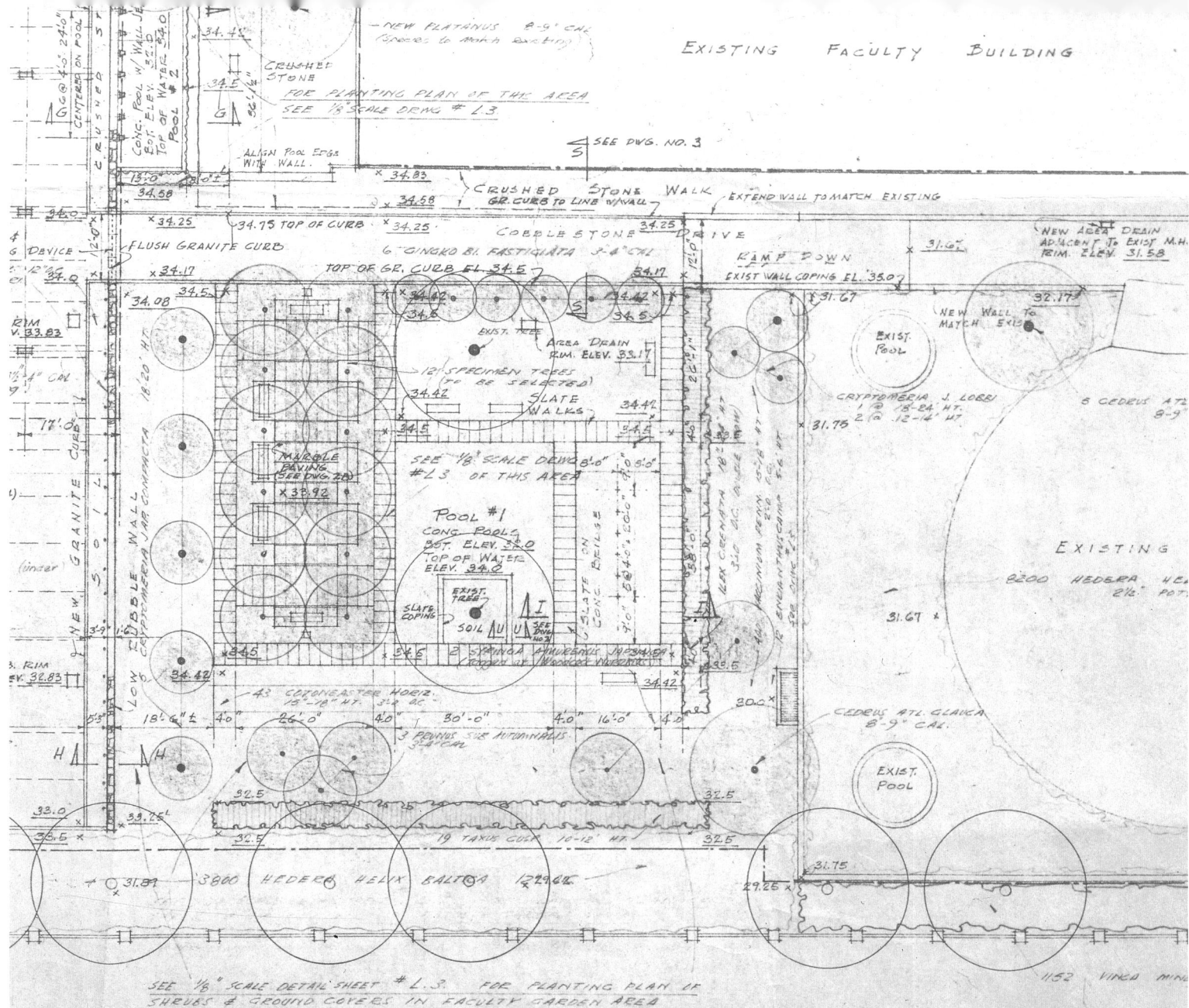

This detail of Dan Kiley's landscape plan shows the Philosopher's Garden, outside the Faculty and Students Club.

The campus of old and new buildings was knitted together through a landscape design by Dan Kiley, the renowned American landscape architect. Taking advantage of an existing line of London plane trees and the Beaux Arts layout of the original campus, Kiley strove to create an urban oasis that would protect and soothe its inhabitants. Today the landscape remains true in spirit to Kiley's design, with plantings added in 1994 during a restoration of the gardens. At that time, while Torsten Wiesel was president, the University also renovated the interiors of Caspary Auditorium and the Abby Aldrich Rockefeller Hall.

The interior of Abby Aldrich Rockefeller Hall c. 1960.

In the 1950s, with the graduate program under way and new facilities completed, Bronk set about expanding the faculty. As he strengthened the traditional biomedical areas of research, Bronk added faculty members whose interests he believed to be part of the working vocabulary of every broadly educated scientist. Biologist Paul Weiss, geneticist Edward Tatum (who would win a Nobel Prize in 1958), and biochemist and Nobel laureate Fritz Lipmann came to Rockefeller.

Bronk gave the Institute instant status in physics by recruiting researchers with international reputations. In 1961 George Uhlenbeck, Ted Berlin, and Mark Kac joined the Institute, bringing complementary interests in theoretical physics and mathematics. Physicist Abraham Pais became a member of the faculty in 1963, and Nicola Khuri joined his group in 1964. Bronk also planned a program in philosophy at Rockefeller, bringing in Ludwig Edelstein as professor. To develop research in the behavioral sciences, in 1965 he hired Carl Pfaffmann, who was made a vice president as well as professor. And in 1965 and 1966, Donald Griffin and Peter Marler joined the faculty to initiate studies on animal behavior in collaboration with the New York Zoological Society. Several years later the University acquired land near Millbrook, New York, and established the Center for Field Research in Ethology and Ecology.

Bronk's academic philosophy pushed Rockefeller into new territory, but it also was in accord with the Institute's past. The Institute had always been a federation of laboratories, undivided by departmental or disciplinary boundaries. Although many of the new faculty held similar research interests, Bronk took care not to hire groups of scientists who might function as university departments. Instead he fostered his ideal of a unity of knowledge.

"The growth of knowledge and the increase of information regarding man and nature encourages specialization," Bronk wrote. "But understanding requires comprehension of many related fields of learning." To further round out the disciplines represented on campus, Bronk invited researchers from other institutions for short appointments as visiting professors. And to ensure that Rockefeller's scientists would get to know each other's work, Bronk inaugurated the Friday afternoon lecture series, which in its early years featured only speakers from the faculty.

During Bronk's administration the University also reached out to younger audiences for Rockefeller science. In homage to the tradition of Christmas lectures at the Royal Society in London, Rockefeller biochemist Alfred E. Mirsky founded a similar series for high school students in 1959, and they continue today. René Dubos delivered the first of these lectures.

Unraveling Antibodies

Rockefeller was founded for the study of infectious diseases. Almost since that time researchers here also have focused on the human body's means for responding to disease—the immune system. Henry Kunkel, who came to the Rockefeller Hospital in 1947, studied diseases such as lupus erythematosus and rheumatoid arthritis, in which the immune system attacks the patient's own body. Kunkel's laboratory advanced basic biological knowledge of antibodies, the body's key chemical defenders against infectious organisms.

Kunkel, who died in 1983, was also a remarkable teacher. He trained dozens of researchers, one of whom—Gerald Edelman—went on to win a Nobel Prize in 1972 for determining the complete chemical structure of an antibody. Edelman received his Ph.D. from Rockefeller in 1960 and joined the faculty that year.

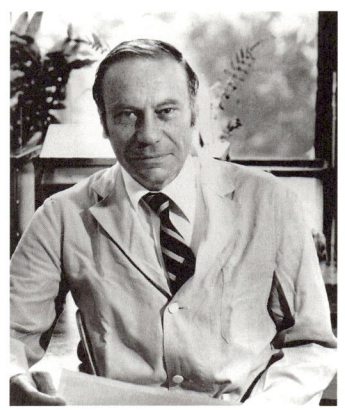

Immunologist Henry Kunkel in 1973.

Mathematician Mark Kac delivered the Mirsky Lecture for high school students in 1962.

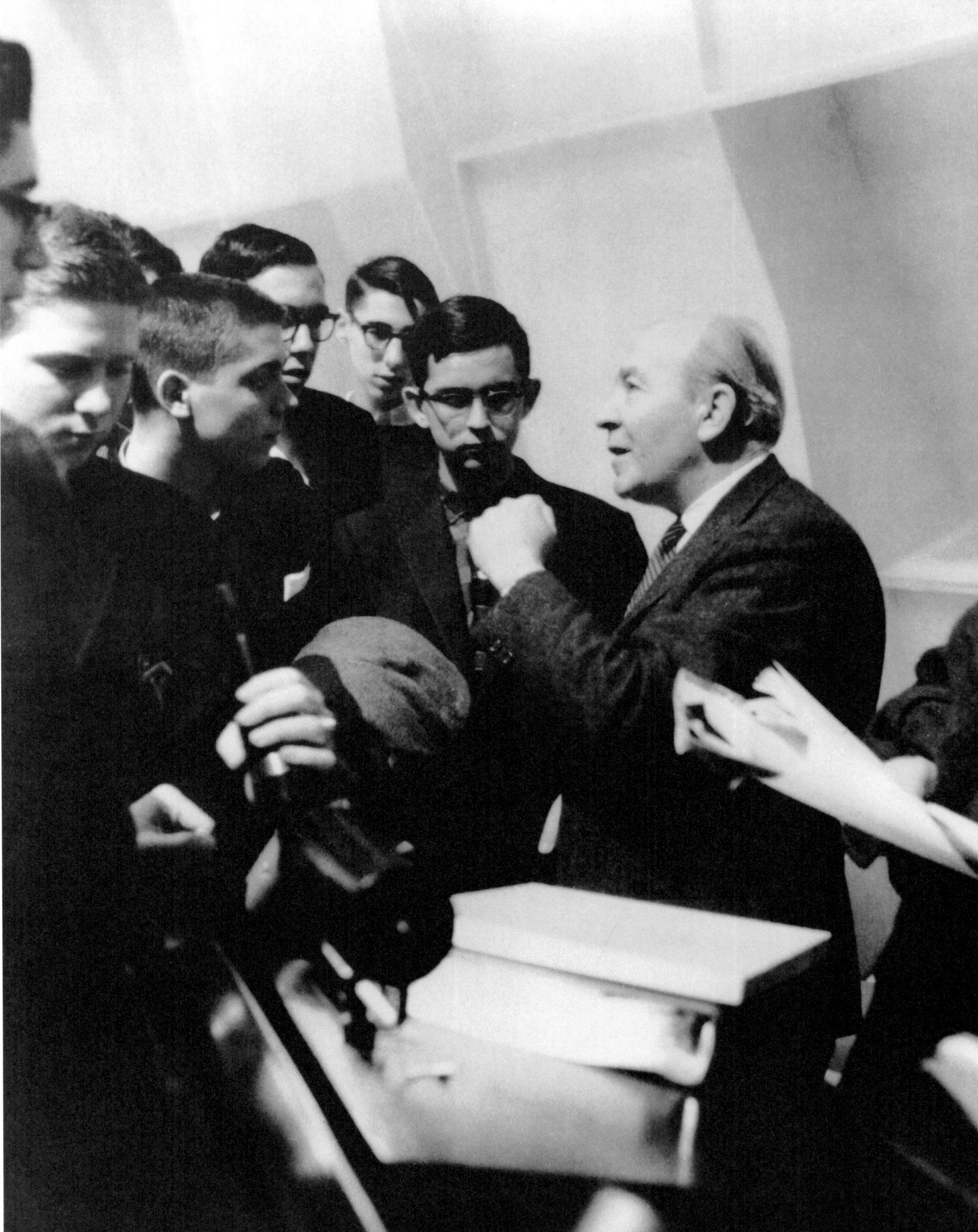

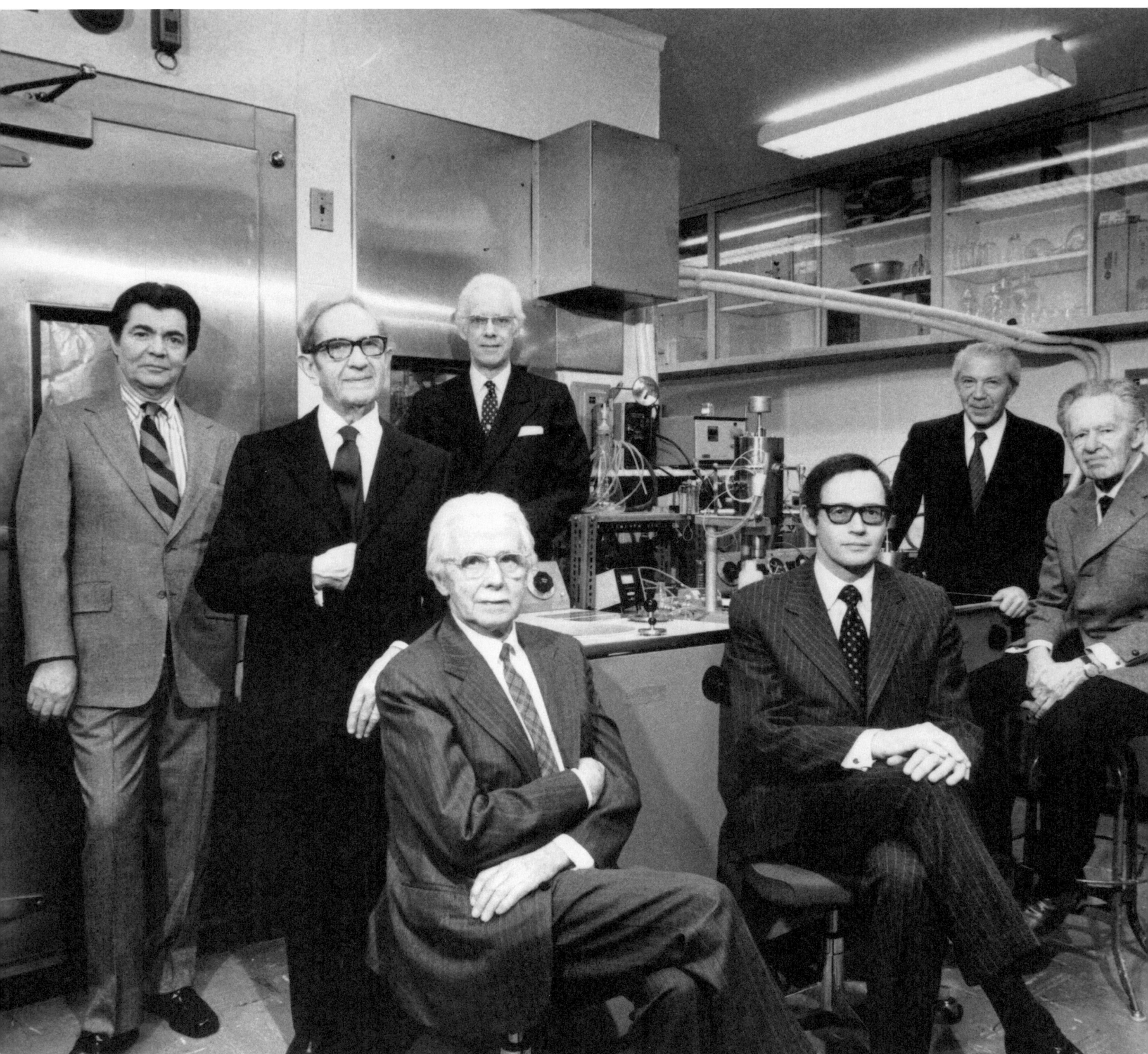

When Bronk retired in 1968 he left behind a University transformed. The number of faculty and staff had tripled, and more than 100 graduate students pursued their degrees here. Rockefeller presidents had traditionally held absolute power over University affairs, but under Bronk a reappraisal of this structure began. Bronk created a Senate of tenured faculty, and in 1967 an Academic Council was elected from the Senate to act as a steering committee and advise the president. Finally, whereas the Institute had previously operated within the means of its endowment income, during Bronk's administration the scientific staff for the first time procured grants from federal agencies to fund research. The 15 years of Bronk's presidency were a time of expansion and optimism for science in the United States generally. The activities at Rockefeller reflected these prosperous times.

Frederick Seitz, a renowned solid state physicist, former president of the National Academy of Sciences and member of the Rockefeller Board of Trustees, became the University's next president. While the transformation from Institute to University had created much to praise, it had also strained financial resources. Seitz took quick steps to stabilize the University's finances. Some measures, such as terminating the philosophy program, were inevitably unpopular and raised questions about the viability of Bronk's initiatives. Managing the University's budget remained a continuous challenge through the 1970s, first because the federal government cut research grants and later because of steep inflation. More funding was clearly needed, and in 1971 Seitz launched the University's first development campaign to systematically seek private support outside the Rockefeller family.

The University continued to be a center of scientific excellence. Seitz recalls that when he became president, Peyton Rous reminded him, "there is no need for anyone here to do anything trivial." Rockefeller faculty were not under the same pressure as other academics to publish or perish. The significance of Rockefeller research was acknowledged with six Nobel Prizes awarded to faculty members and alumni during Seitz's administration. Seitz also nurtured scientific talent at Rockefeller in new ways, launching the M.D.-Ph.D. program in collaboration with Cornell University Medical College. And during his administration Seitz successfully completed several building projects on campus—the Tower building (now the Benjamin and Irma G. Weiss Research Building), the Laboratory Animal Research Center, and the Faculty House apartments.

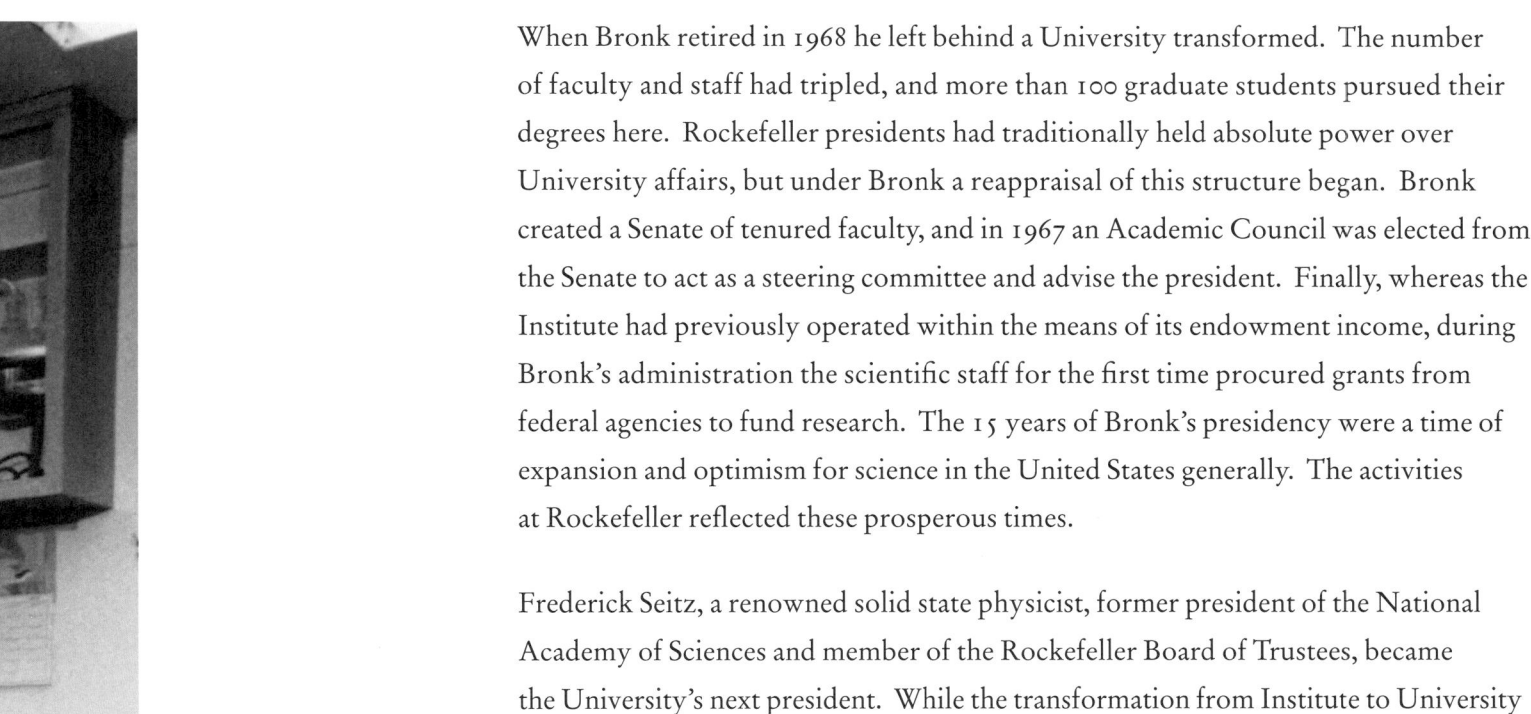

Seven Rockefeller Nobel laureates posed for this photograph in 1976. Standing, from left: George Palade, Albert Claude, Stanford Moore, Christian de Duve. Seated, from left: H. Keffer Hartline, Gerald Edelman, Fritz Lipmann.

During the 1970s the tools of molecular biology became increasingly important in the study of life processes and the underlying causes of disease. Progress in mapping human chromosomes was leading to a deeper knowledge of genetic disorders, cancer, and aging. At the same time, the use of computers transformed the practice of science. Joshua Lederberg, who served as president of Rockefeller from 1978 to 1990, held widespread interests that uniquely qualified him to lead the University at this pivotal time. A Nobel laureate for his work on the organization of genetic material in bacteria, Lederberg had been a professor of both biology and computer science at Stanford University, as well as head of its Department of Genetics.

Lederberg brought several new faculty to the University during his tenure as president. By the 1970s Rockefeller had grown to about 50 laboratories, with long-established professors heading groups of up to 50 scientists and staff working under them. To sustain its leadership in science, the University needed to recruit a new generation of investigators. Lederberg created research opportunities for young scientists, and established new laboratories in biochemical genetics, organic chemistry and biochemistry, plant molecular biology, parasitology, the biology of skin diseases, neurobiology, and neurochemistry. An agreement forged with the Howard Hughes Medical Institute in 1986 initiated the construction of a new laboratory building on campus and the hiring of joint Rockefeller-HHMI faculty. The rejuvenation of the faculty that Lederberg set in motion has been the most significant change in the University's structure in recent decades.

The policy of recruiting young scientists to the faculty accelerated through the brief presidency of Rockefeller alumnus and Nobel laureate David Baltimore, from 1990 to 1992, and in particular under the leadership of Torsten Wiesel. Wiesel, who received a Nobel Prize for studies of how visual information is transmitted to the brain and who has been a member of the Rockefeller faculty since 1983, was president of the University from 1992 to 1998. In that interval 30 new laboratories were established at the University and, for the first time, laboratories headed by untenured faculty were created.

"These new faculty members have had a profound effect on academic life here at Rockefeller," says Wiesel. "They have created a renewed sense of intellectual and scientific vitality." Wiesel also inaugurated six research centers, which facilitate

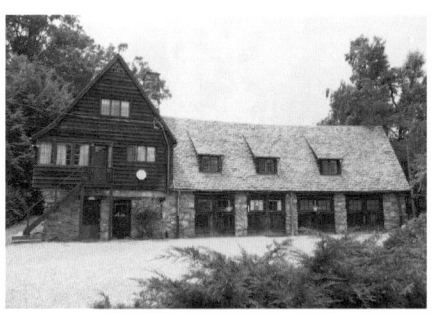

The Center for Field Research in Ethology and Ecology in Millbrook, New York. Fernando Nottebohm directs the Center today.

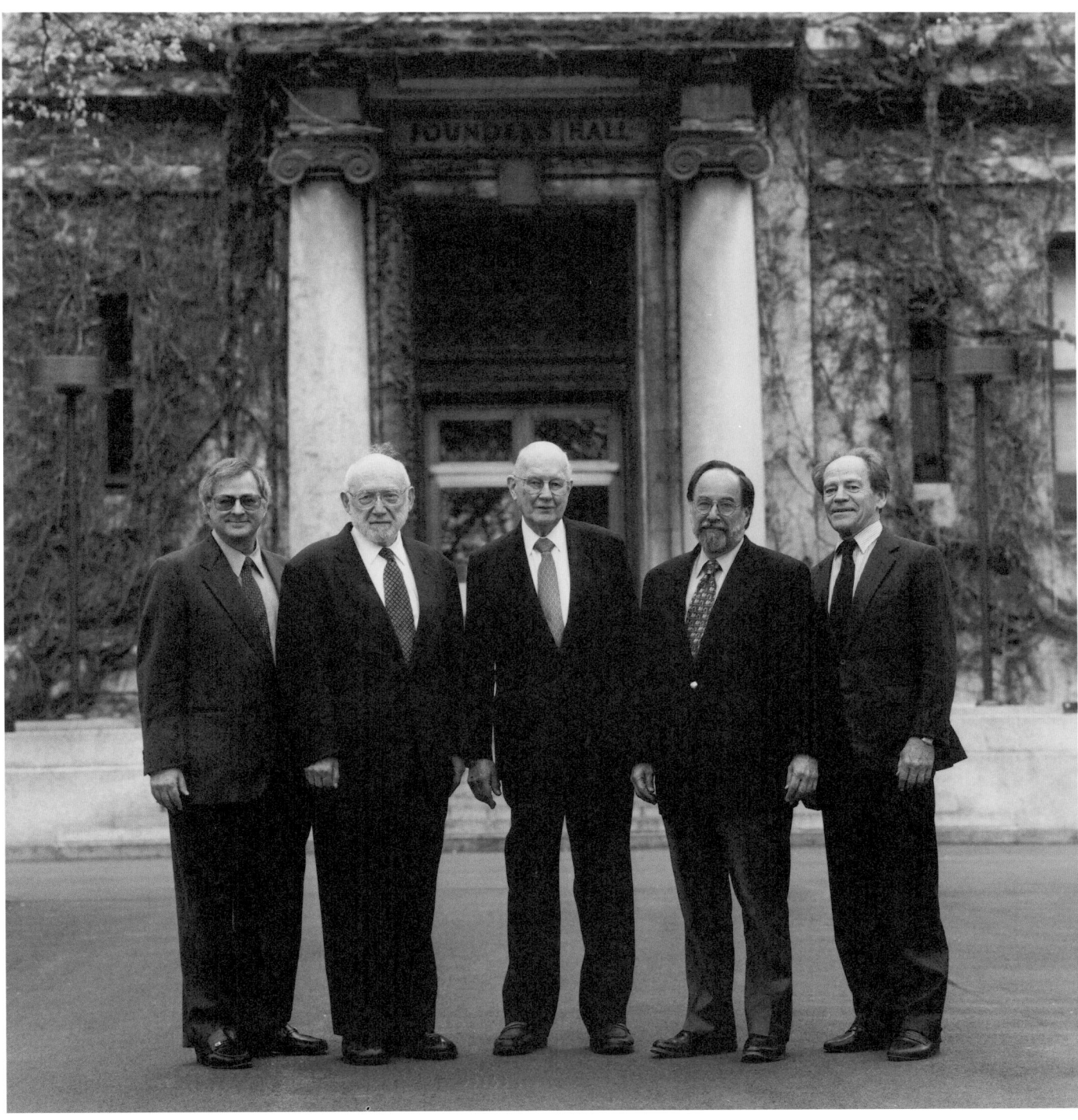

The five most recent presidents of The Rockefeller University, photographed in 1999. From left to right: Arnold J. Levine, Joshua Lederberg, Frederick Seitz, David Baltimore, Torsten N. Wiesel.

collaboration among University faculty working in similar areas without the administrative apparatus of formal departments. Notably, Wiesel achieved all of this while setting the University on a course of fiscal and institutional stability.

Arnold Levine, a renowned cancer biologist, became the eighth president of Rockefeller in December 1998. He holds great respect for the history of this place—a past that guides its future. "The integrity of the University's founders—their commitment to excellence, to freedom of inquiry, and to keeping the place intimate and collegial—has consistently fostered great science," says Levine. This well-established formula for success continues to serve Rockefeller in its second century. "Novel interdisciplinary approaches have always found favor at Rockefeller," Levine adds, "and the future of science depends on defying accepted scientific boundaries." Adding new faculty in key fields, encouraging greater collaboration among researchers, modernizing the University's research hospital, and enhancing the graduate program and public education are steps Levine is taking to lead Rockefeller's scientists to future success.

GROWTH

A Closer Look: From Institute to University

The "Charter Class" 100

Viruses, Cancer, and Perseverance 102

Hope for Heroin Addicts 105

Investigating Heart Disease and Obesity 106

Unpacking Proteins 108

The Henry Ford of Protein Synthesis 111

Shaping Science Policy 112

The "Charter Class"

Lee D. Peachey was a member of Rockefeller's first class of Ph.D.'s, graduating in 1959. For most of his subsequent career he has been professor of biology at the University of Pennsylvania, a position from which he retired in 2000. On the occasion of The Rockefeller University's centennial, he shares his recollections of the interview with Detlev Bronk that gained him admission to the "Charter Class":

"Bronk greeted me, shook my hand, and started talking. He told me about the student program, and how it wasn't like other, ordinary graduate programs. His goal was to educate the whole person, not just the technically qualified, to take his/her place in society and in the world….Bronk read me letters from leading scientists all over the world (all close friends of his), including one in French from Monod (I didn't understand a word, but I tried to look knowledgeable and impressed). He told me about his plans to bring students into contact with leaders in the artistic world as part of their training experience, and his desire that all students would spend a year abroad with one or another of the famous scientists with which he was in close contact (more letters read, and *lots* of names dropped). There were to be no courses as such, but only direct contact for extended periods with the great people who had actually done the great works. This went on for well over an hour…

"Around noon, by which time I had not said a single word, Bronk sat back and said that he had become convinced that I was not one of those undesirables who wanted only narrow technical training (probably not his exact words), and that in fact I was 'just the sort of person he wanted' in his program (I think those *were* his exact words). I remember trying to say something, and having to clear my throat first, as I had been silent for so long that the words wouldn't come out. I reassured him that I was interested in just the kind of training he was describing,…and that was it: I had been accepted…

The five graduates at the first Convocation in 1959 receiving congratulations from chairman of the board David Rockefeller and president Detlev Bronk. From left: William F. Arndt Jr., Suydam Osterhout, David Rockefeller, Detlev Bronk, Lee D. Peachey, Harold J. Simon, Howard Rasmussen.

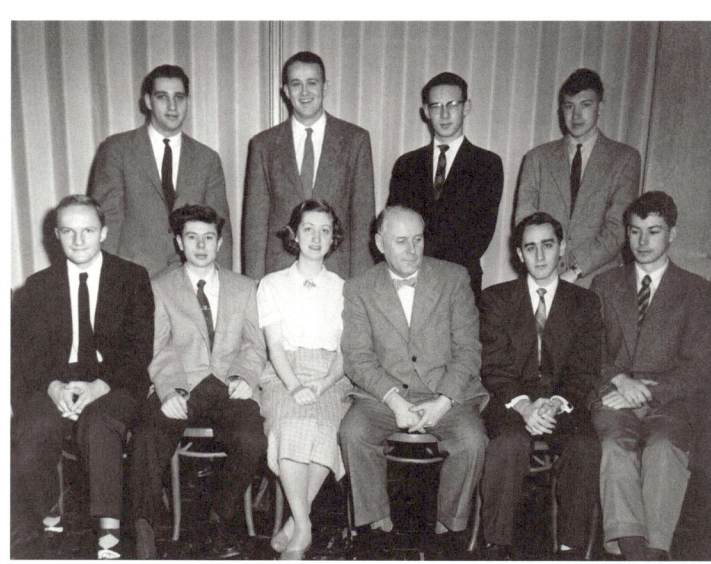

Members of the first class of graduate students entering Rockefeller, with visiting scientist Ragnar Granit, who shared a Nobel Prize with H. Keffer Hartline. Standing, from left: Lewis J. Greene, Allen B. Edmundson, Frederick A. Dodge Jr., Johns W. Hopkins III. Seated, from left: Donald A. Young, John J. Cebra, Mary A. Bonneville, Ragnar Granit, Sanford A. Lacks, Eystein K.M. Paasche. Not shown is William F. Arndt Jr.

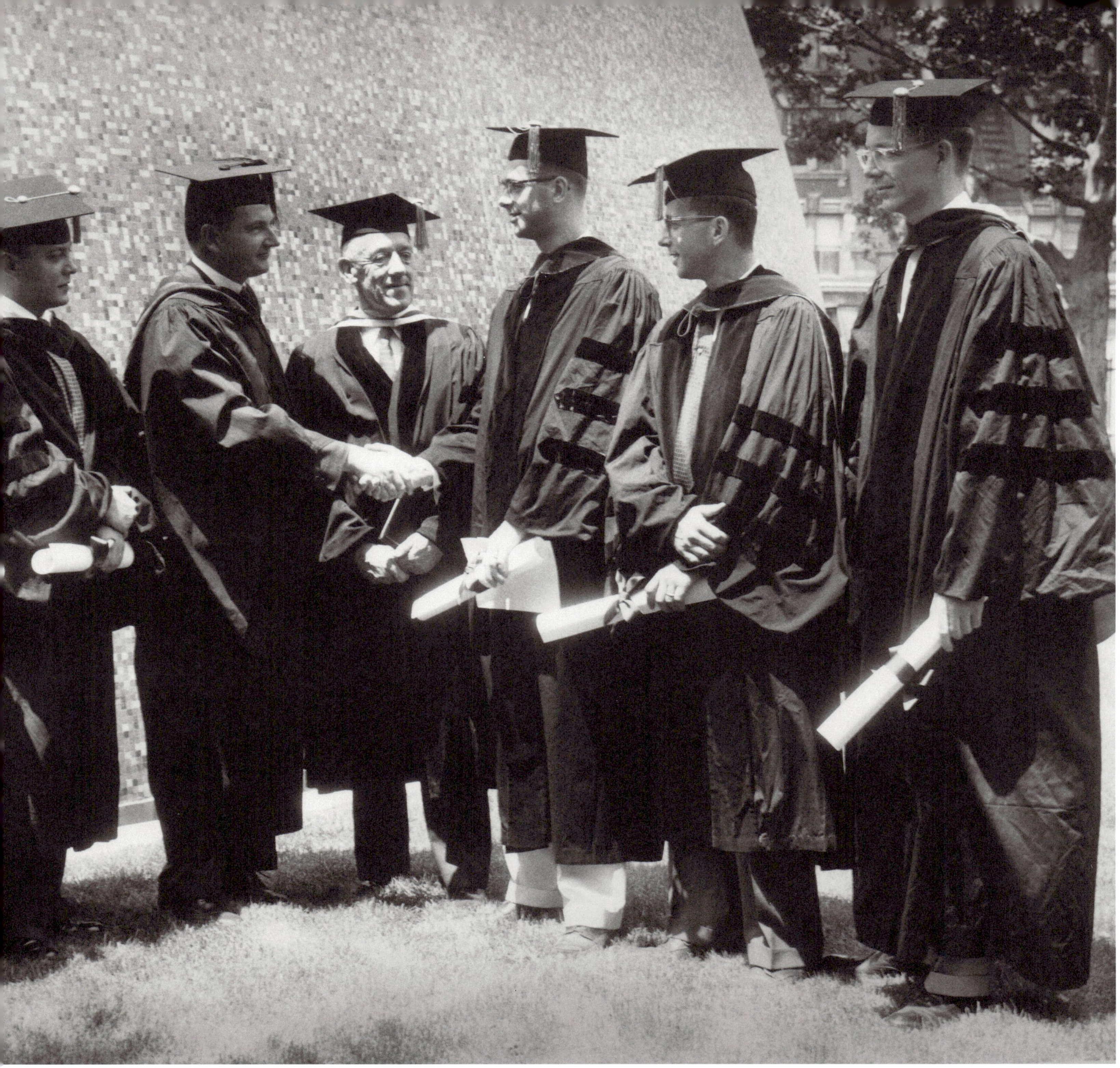

"Lest I give the impression that I was not impressed with Bronk or that I am not extremely grateful for the opportunities and education he made possible for me, let me say that his graduate program *did* turn out to be special in many ways. He made good on his promises to bring us up against a lot of great people, both in science and in the arts and other fields such as publishing. We did have dinners and evenings with people like the head of the Museum of Modern Art and the science editor of the *New York Times*. We received lectures from a long series of very distinguished scientists, mostly Nobel laureates, all of whom stayed a week or even two and who spent big parts of those days with us, often including dinner and evenings together. True, they often had been given little or no advance idea of what we already knew or what or who had come before. On occasion we even had to ask the speaker his name, as we were given no advance schedule. Every Monday morning we had a surprise. Some of these weeks were disasters, but many were priceless. Clearly, we, the students, were very special to Dr. Bronk, and we were treated like the chosen ones. And we loved it!"

Viruses, Cancer, and Perseverance

In 1966 Peyton Rous received a Nobel Prize for his discovery that a virus can cause cancer. It was an acknowledgment spectacularly deferred: Rous had published his discovery in 1911, just two years after he defied the advice of his mentor, William Welch, and came to The Rockefeller Institute to study cancer. In 1911 the world of science was not ready to accept such a startling assertion. Nevertheless Rous persisted in his research, and in the intervening years the virus known as the Rous sarcoma virus became an essential tool for investigating the cellular mechanisms that go awry in cancer.

Rous found the virus in the tumor of a chicken—a barred Plymouth Rock hen with a growth on her right breast. A poultry breeder had noticed the large lump and brought the hen to The Rockefeller Institute. The tumor was a sarcoma, an abnormal growth of cells of the connective tissue. To test the possibility that it was caused by an infectious agent, Rous prepared an extract—he minced a sample of the tumor tissue in a liquid solution and passed this through a filter to eliminate bacteria and tumor cells. Then he injected the extract into healthy chickens. Contrary to his expectations, it produced new tumors. Describing these experiments, Rous suggested that the tumor-inducing agent was "a minute parasitic organism"—a virus.

At the time, viruses were poorly understood, and few scientists believed that cancer could be caused by an infection. In the early 1930s Rous pursued further evidence for viral causes of cancer. A colleague at Rockefeller, Richard Shope, discovered that a mammalian tumor—a papilloma, or wart—found in rabbits was caused by a virus. Rous conducted studies with it, keeping alive the viral theory of cancer causation. But it was a new generation of biologists, using the methods of molecular biology, who unraveled the explanation for the ability of Rous sarcoma virus to transform normal cells into cancerous ones.

In the 1950s the virus became a tool for studying cancer because—unlike chemicals or radiation—it reliably and reproducibly induced tumors. Harry Rubin and Howard Temin at the California Institute of Technology developed ways to study the virus in tissue culture rather than animals and to analyze its action on cells in terms of chemistry and genetics. In the 1960s a gene called *src* was identified as producing the protein that leads to tumors.

Although much of the ensuing research on *src* has been done elsewhere, the Rockefeller connection to the Rous sarcoma virus has remained strong. Beginning in the 1970s Hidesaburo Hanafusa, who had worked in Temin's laboratory, investigated the genetics of the virus. More recently, several laboratories at Rockefeller have collaborated to understand the structure of the protein produced by *src*. In 1997 the laboratory of John Kuriyan published the three-dimensional structure of the protein, a structure that reveals how the molecule functions.

Decades of work on the Rous sarcoma virus also have been important because the virus belongs to a group known as retroviruses, which includes the virus that causes AIDS. Basic knowledge gleaned from studies of the Rous sarcoma virus enabled researchers to find ways of treating AIDS much more quickly than otherwise would have been possible.

In addition to his discovery of a cancer-causing virus, Peyton Rous is remembered for developing a method for preserving whole blood for transfusion, and for the high standards of scientific exposition he maintained during more than four decades as an editor of The Journal of Experimental Medicine.

By injecting this hen with a filtered extract that contained a virus, Rous induced a tumor to form (below). (c. 1911)

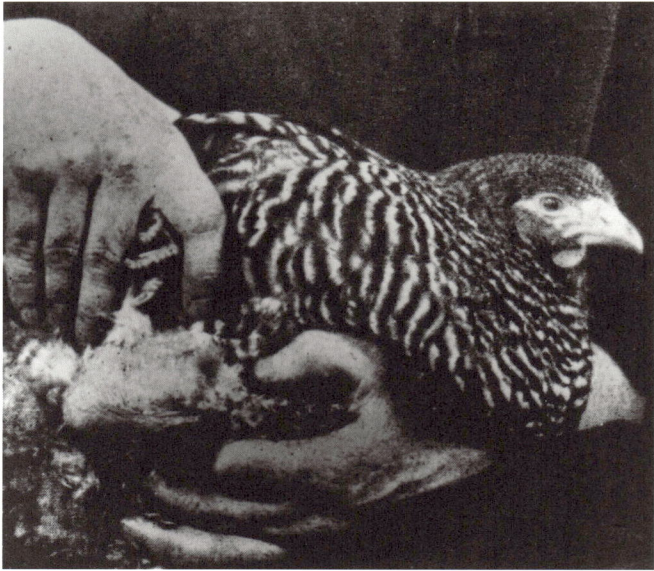

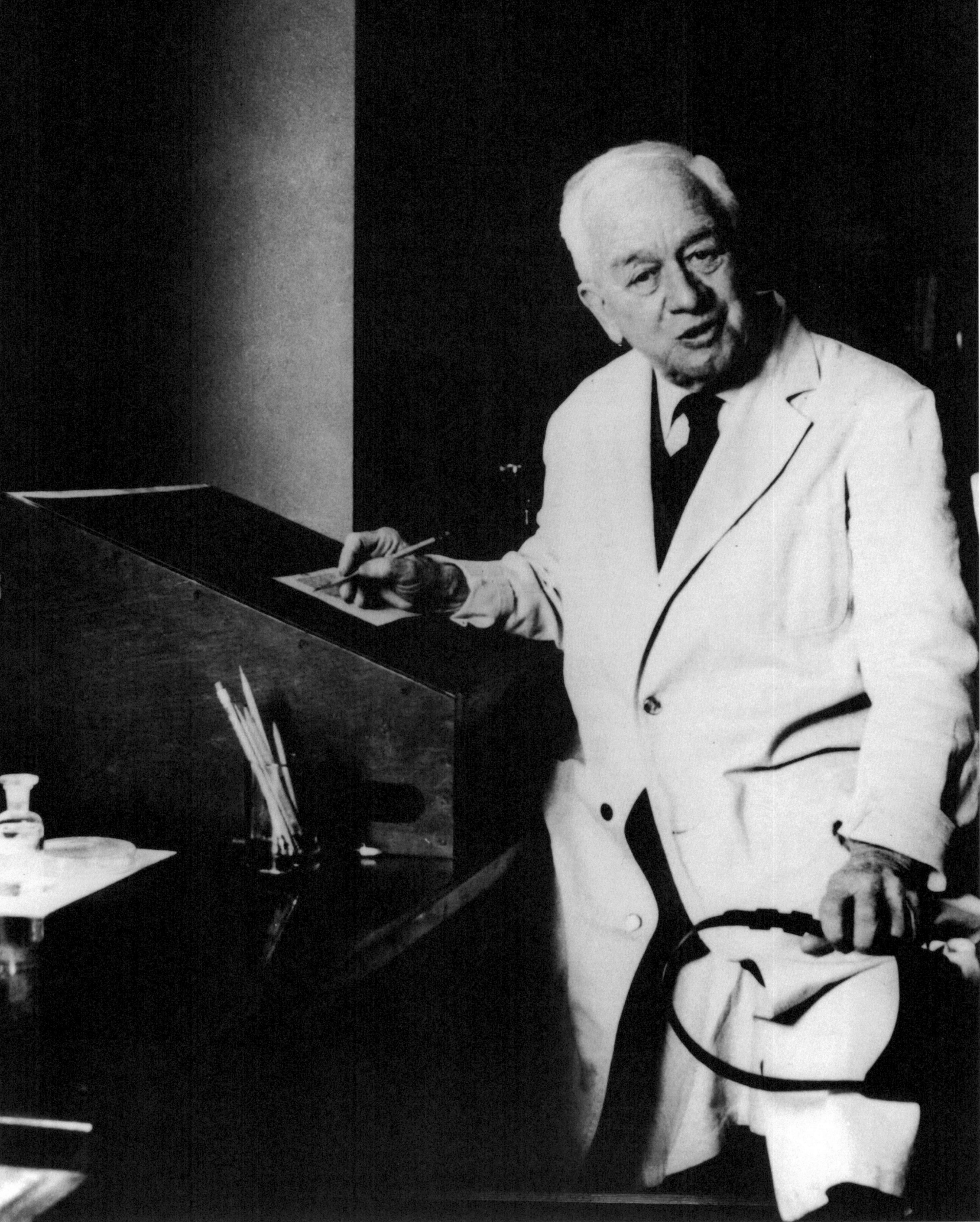

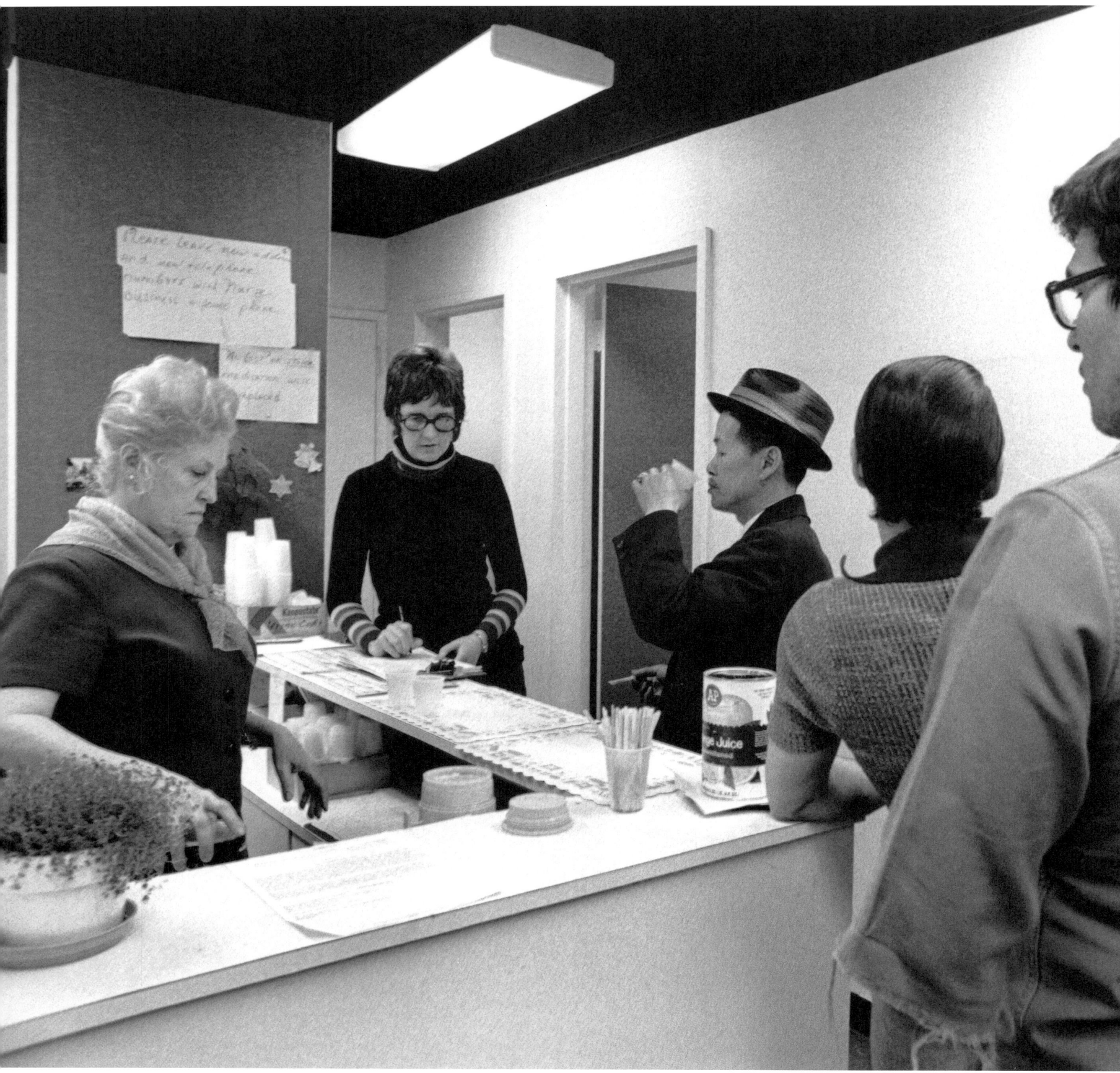

Research on heroin addiction at the Rockefeller Hospital led to methadone maintenance clinics like this one at Beth Israel Hospital in New York City. (1972)

Hope for Heroin Addicts

Heroin abuse surged in the United States in the 1960s. Most people at the time assumed that drug addiction was the fault of the addict—a personal moral failing, lack of willpower, or simply criminal behavior. But Vincent Dole, now professor emeritus, wondered if there might be a different explanation. Could addiction be explained in terms of a chemical imbalance—a misfire of metabolism?

It was an idea that followed from Dole's experience in the laboratory of pioneering clinical chemist Donald Van Slyke, where he came to work in 1941. Later, in his own laboratory, he studied the biochemistry of metabolic disorders such as hypertension and obesity. A year spent as chairman of the New York City Health Department's committee on narcotics in the early 1960s convinced Dole that heroin addiction, in addition to being a social problem, was a disorder deserving medical treatment. In 1964 he teamed up with Marie Nyswander, a psychiatrist who had been working with addicts since the 1940s, and Mary Jeanne Kreek, an assistant resident at New York Hospital, now New York Presbyterian.

To figure out how to get addicts off heroin, Dole and Nyswander first set out to test the way the body processes different narcotics. Rockefeller president Detlev Bronk gave them permission to admit six heroin addicts to the Rockefeller Hospital for the study. It was a decision that might have provoked controversy or even harassment, given the social stigma of addiction and the fact that parts of the study required giving some addicts heroin to compare its effects with other narcotics and, later, its interaction with methadone. As it happened, no trouble ensued. Dole attributes this largely to Bronk's support of the project.

Along with other narcotics, Dole and Nyswander tested methadone, a synthetic drug developed in Germany during World War II as an analgesic to replace morphine. So long as the addicts took methadone, heroin had no effect on them, nor did they crave it. Methadone was not a cure for addiction—the addicts needed a daily maintenance dose—but it allowed them to function relatively normally. With methadone they could go back to work and reconcile family relationships strained by their heroin habits.

Building on this success, the researchers carried out expanded studies at Beth Israel Medical Center. Methadone maintenance was soon made available to tens of thousands of addicts in New York and other cities. In 1971 Dole introduced methadone to the Manhattan House of Detention for Men—popularly called "The Tombs"—to detoxify heroin addicts in the overcrowded prison.

Dole later extended his work on the biochemical effects of addictive substances and carried out studies of alcoholism. Addiction research continues at Rockefeller today in the laboratory headed by Mary Jeanne Kreek, whose work focuses on understanding the biological basis of opiate addiction, cocaine dependency, and alcoholism.

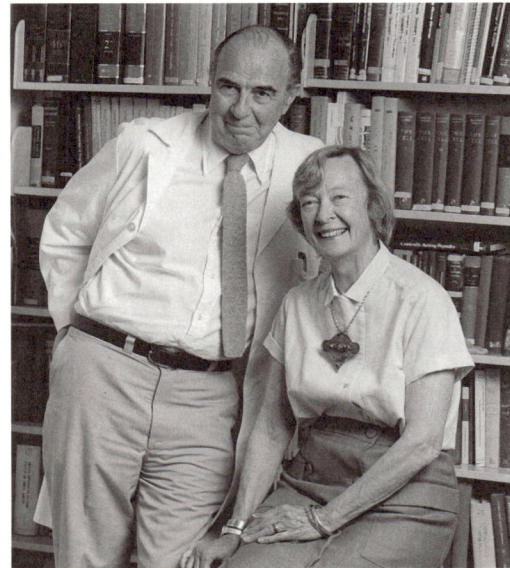

Vincent Dole and Marie Nyswander teamed up in the mid-1960s to study the chemical nature of heroin addiction.

Investigating Heart Disease and Obesity

Cholesterol, diet, heart disease, and obesity are interrelated in complex ways in the human body. For more than a half century clinical researchers at the Rockefeller Hospital have sought to unravel these relationships. Their groundbreaking results include the finding that unsaturated fat can lower cholesterol, the elucidation of a "set point" mechanism by which the human body tends to maintain a stable weight, and the discovery of genes that play important roles in heart disease and obesity.

Understanding metabolism has provided one approach to the problems of heart disease and obesity. In the 1940s scientists were beginning to find evidence that fat in the diet plays a role in atherosclerosis—the buildup of fatty compounds like cholesterol on the inner walls of arteries that can lead to heart attack. But few details were known about how the body processes and uses fat in food. Vincent Dole made an important advance in this knowledge when he devised a way to measure energy-transporting compounds called free fatty acids in the blood. It was a step toward a chemical understanding of how fat is metabolized.

Edward H. Ahrens Jr. developed this line of research further. In the early 1950s he became the first to do careful dietary studies, using formula diets, to test the effects of different types of fats on cholesterol levels. To carry out these studies it was necessary to chemically separate the different types of fat, called lipids, circulating in the blood. Jules Hirsch collaborated on this project when he joined Ahrens' laboratory at the Rockefeller Hospital in 1954.

While Ahrens focused on heart disease, Hirsch soon became interested in understanding obesity. His research has led to many important findings, including the discovery that obese people have much larger adipocytes, or fat cells, than individuals of normal weight and that some obese people also have significantly more fat cells. Hirsch points out that understanding human problems like heart disease and obesity has been Rockefeller's mission from its founding. It is "the glory of the place," he says, that clinical understanding of these disorders has led to important scientific results.

While metabolic studies continued, researchers in the 1980s began applying the tools of molecular biology and genetics to the study of heart disease and obesity. Jan L. Breslow came to Rockefeller in 1984 to study the hereditary component of atherosclerosis.

Breslow and his coworkers have found one gene in particular that can predispose a person to atherosclerosis. It controls the level of a substance in the blood known as apolipoprotein E, which ferries cholesterol through the bloodstream.

Obesity and related disorders such as heart disease and diabetes are the research focus of Rockefeller alumnus Jeffrey Friedman, who joined the faculty in 1986. Friedman, who is also a Howard Hughes Medical Investigator, has gained international recognition for the discovery of an obesity-regulating gene and its protein product, the weight-regulating hormone leptin.

Scientists inject DNA into mouse embryos in order to study how the new genes function in living animals. Jan Breslow has developed several such mouse models for research on heart disease.

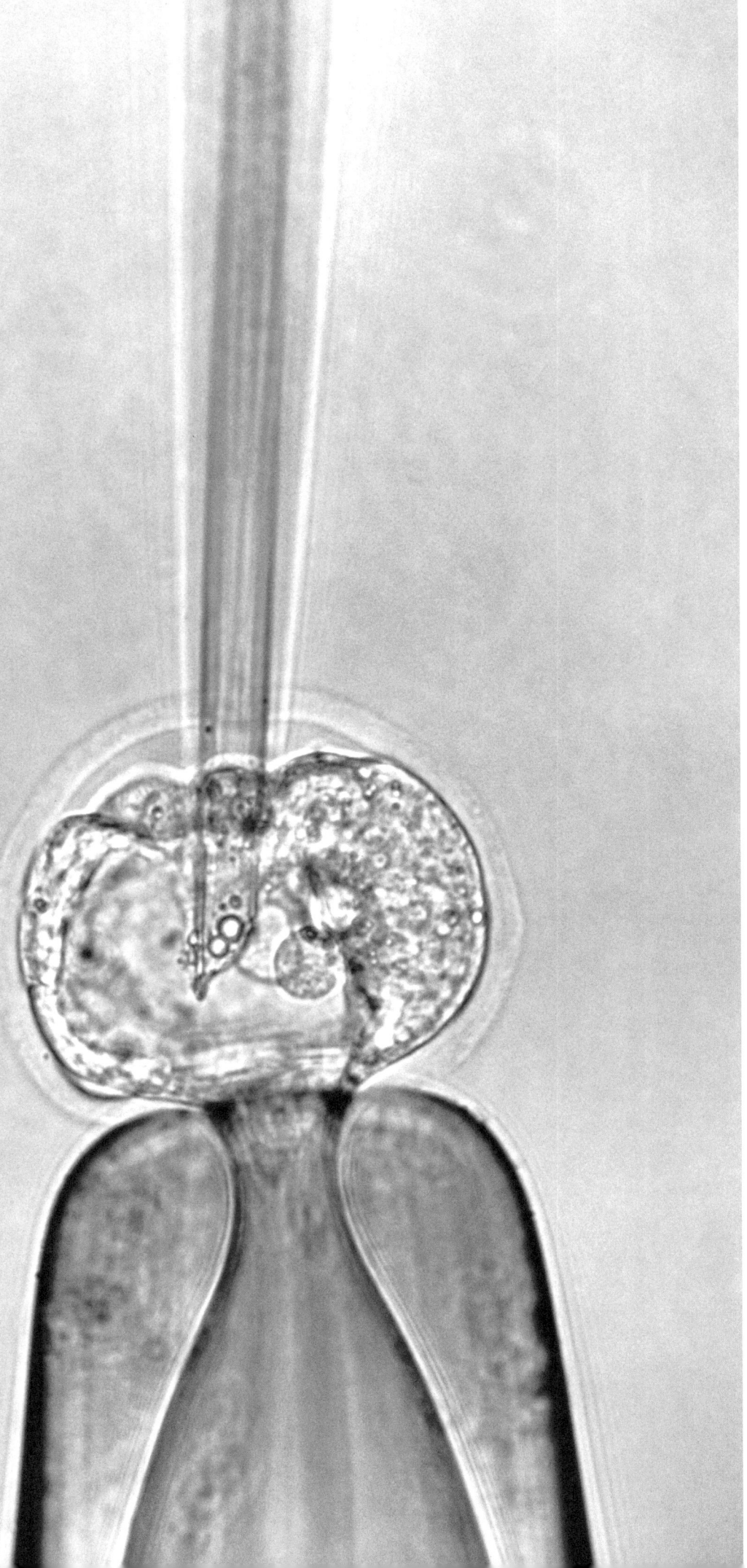

Unpacking Proteins

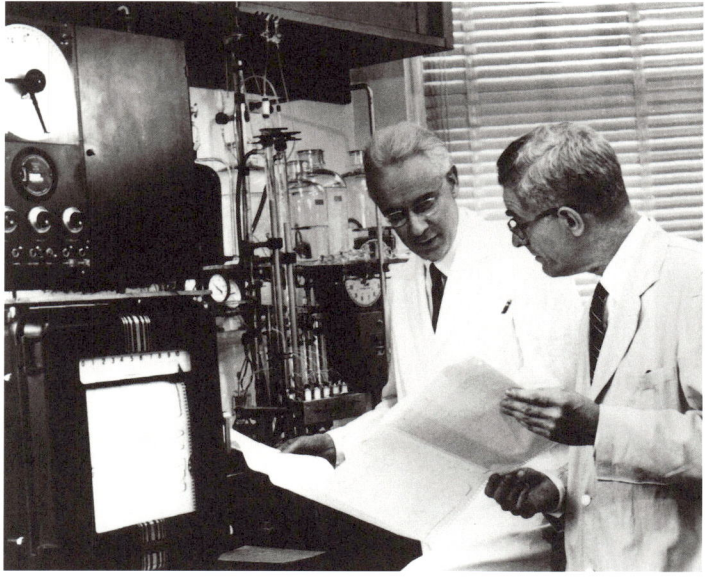

William Stein came to The Rockefeller Institute in 1937 to work in the laboratory of renowned protein chemist Max Bergmann. In 1939 Stanford Moore joined the laboratory, and there began a collaboration that continued later in their own joint laboratory and would last more than 40 years.

Moore and Stein focused on working out the chemical structure of proteins. Proteins are the workhorses of biology. Within the human body hormones, growth factors, antibodies, oxygen carriers, enzymes, and many other essential molecules are proteins. Solving the puzzles of protein structures lies at the heart of understanding cancer, among many illnesses, and developing drugs to intervene.

In the 1940s a new tool, chromatography, became available to chemists. Chromatography provides a way to separate mixtures of molecules in solution into pure samples of each type of molecule. Moore and Stein spent several years developing new chromatographic methods that could separate solutions of amino acids—the building blocks of protein. A protein is in essence a chain of amino acids. If the scientists could chemically remove the amino acid links from a protein one at a time, separating the amino acid from the remaining portion of the protein at each step and identifying it, they would be able to determine the sequence of amino acids that made up the protein.

By 1950 Moore and Stein felt ready to try out their technique on a protein larger than any previously analyzed—bovine pancreatic ribonuclease. As Moore explained in a 1982 interview, "We wanted to take on an enzyme so that when we had the structure worked out we could relate it to the catalytic mechanism—in the case of ribonuclease, its action in speeding the process of digesting RNA."

In addition, there were practical reasons for choosing this protein. It was readily available in large quantities as a by-product of meat processing. And it was also a molecule with a history at Rockefeller—René Dubos had developed a method for purifying it, and Moses Kunitz had isolated it in crystalline form.

In 1959 Moore and Stein worked out the complete chemical structure of ribonuclease, a chain of 124 amino acids folded and joined at four places. It was the largest protein for which a structure was known at the time, and in 1972 they received a Nobel Prize for their work, shared with Christian B. Alfinsen.

Above left: Stanford Moore (left) and William Stein with the amino acid analyzer in 1965. Right: Moore and Stein outside the laboratory.

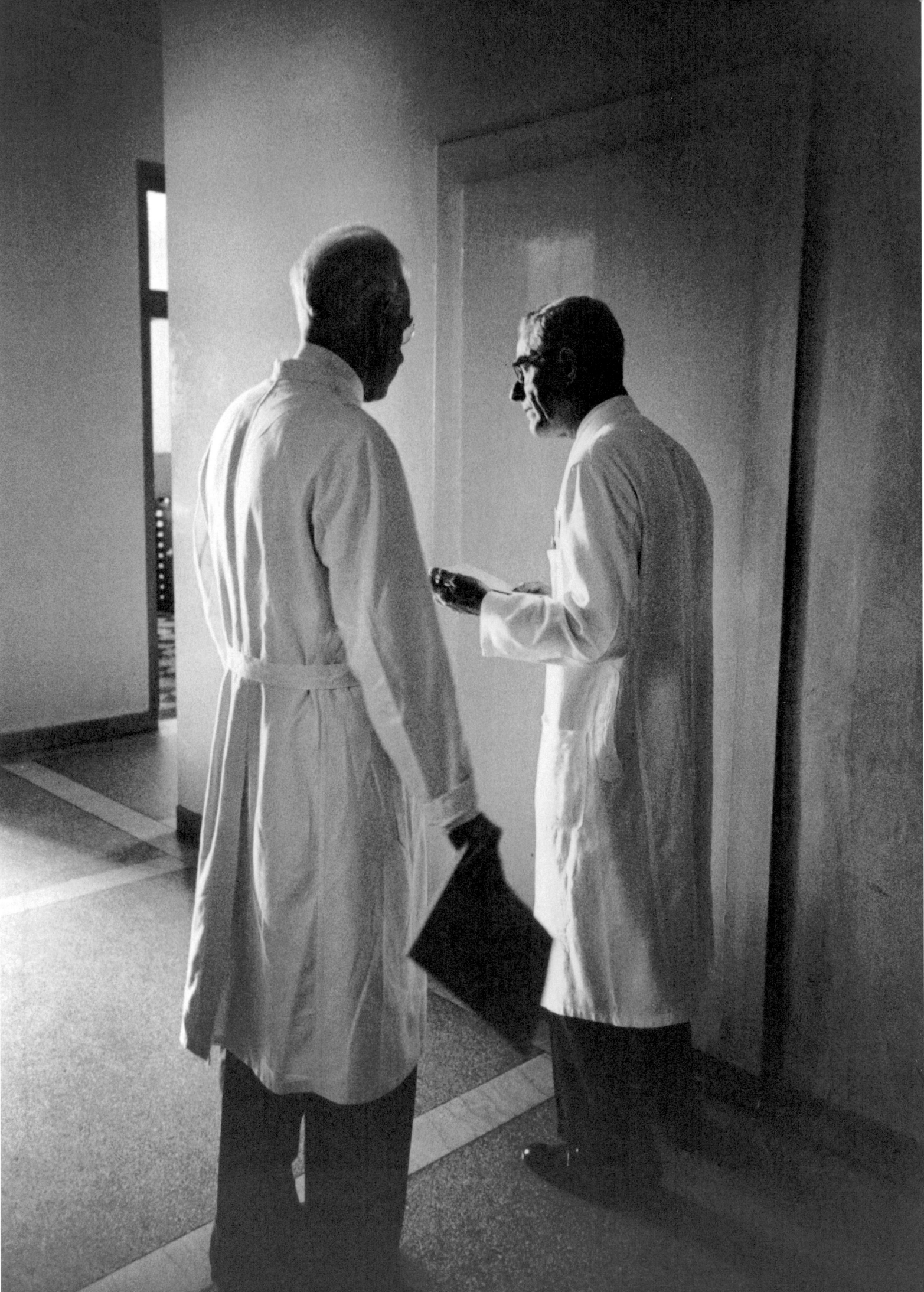

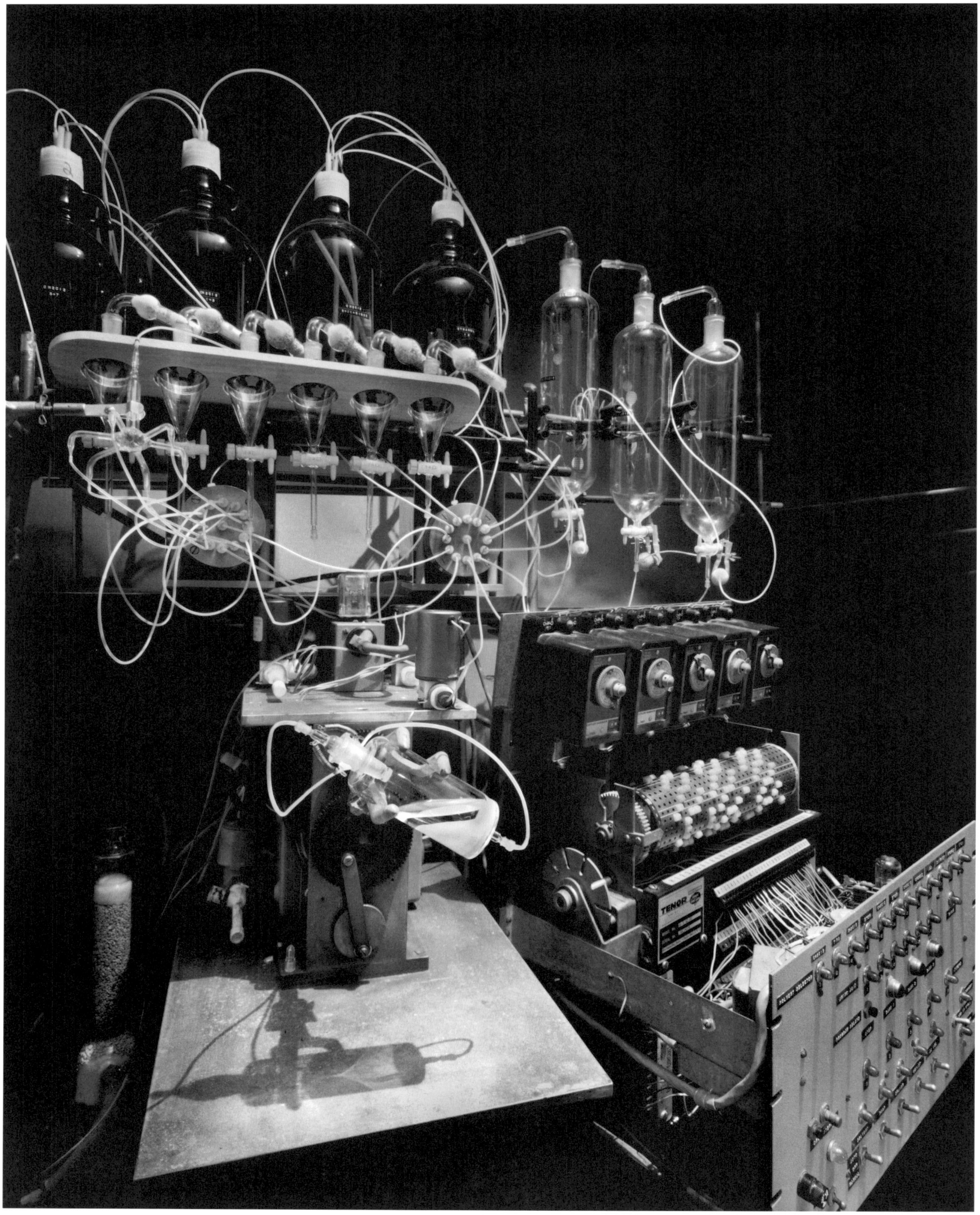

The Henry Ford of Protein Synthesis

Sometimes solving scientific problems requires first inventing the right tool for the job. That was the situation faced by R. Bruce Merrifield in the early 1950s. Working in the Rockefeller laboratory of D. Wayne Woolley, he wanted to synthesize peptides—small versions of proteins—that varied slightly in their structure, so that he could then compare their biological activity. His frustration with this project led him to research that would be honored with a Nobel Prize in 1984.

With the methods of the day, peptide synthesis was a painstaking process. Peptides, like proteins, are chains of amino acid molecules, and the amino acids had to be strung together one at a time in chemical solution. The product was purified after each addition by crystallizing it. Not only was the process time consuming, it also was limited by diminishing returns: the longer the amino acid chain, the more difficult it was to crystallize and the more impurities were present. It required months to hook together a peptide chain of only five amino acids. Synthesizing proteins consisting of hundreds or thousands of amino acids—the interesting ones—was out of the question.

In 1959 Merrifield proposed a solution to this problem: a scaffold of tiny plastic beads to support the growing amino acid chains and eliminate the need for crystallization. He set to work building a prototype, which he estimated he could do in a few months. It took three years to prove the concept and synthesize a nine-amino-acid-long hormone. In the meantime, he had not published a single paper. Merrifield attributes his success in part to Rockefeller's support of such long-term projects without the pressure to publish. "It was extremely important in my case," he says. "If I'd gone as an assistant professor somewhere else and hadn't published, I'd have been out of a job."

After the initial success, Merrifield and colleagues from his laboratory and Rockefeller's instrument shop began automating the process, building a machine that manufactured proteins on an assembly line. By 1965 they had a working model and in 1969 they synthesized ribonuclease—the enzyme whose amino acid sequence had been determined by William H. Stein and Stanford Moore at Rockefeller ten years before. Synthesizing the 124-amino-acid-long enzyme took 369 chemical reactions and 11,391 steps in the machine.

Merrifield's invention, the process called solid-phase peptide synthesis, revolutionized protein chemistry. Now manufactured commercially, peptide synthesizers have since been used to make vaccines, hormones, and a variety of drugs and are standard equipment for research.

An early model of the automated peptide synthesizer (left), and R. Bruce Merrifield, its inventor (below).

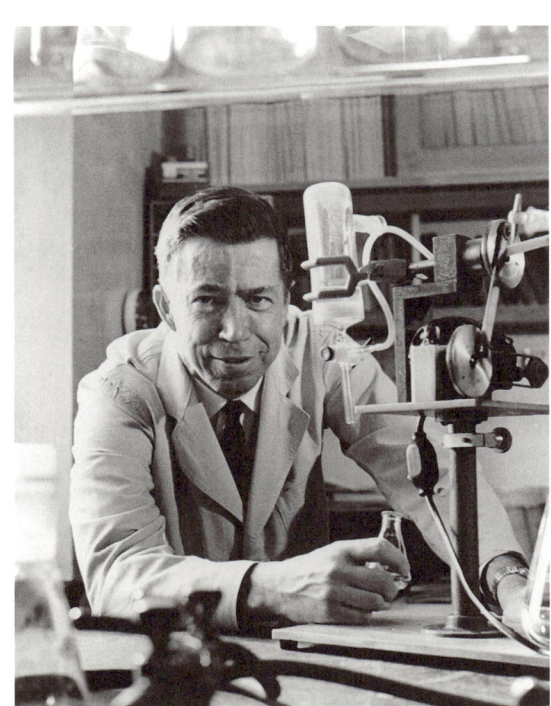

Shaping Science Policy

In the years following World War II, the U.S. federal government began supporting science at unprecedented levels. Detlev Bronk had become well known for his extraordinary administrative talents during the war, through work for the Office of Scientific Research and Development and as special consultant to the Secretary of War. In the 1950s, as government science retooled for the cold war and as the country entered the space age, Bronk became one of the most influential leaders in national science policy.

Bronk, a New Yorker descended from the family for whom the borough of the Bronx is named, was an innovator in science and education as well as policy. He earned his Ph.D. in both physics and physiology in 1926 at the University of Michigan. Working at Cambridge University with E.D. Adrian in 1928, he made the first recording of electrical activity in single nerve fibers. Through this and later research, and during 20 years as director of the Eldridge Reeves Johnson Foundation for Medical Physics at the University of Pennsylvania, Bronk helped establish the discipline of biophysics in the United States. As president of Johns Hopkins University from 1949 to 1953, he sought to remove barriers between undergraduate and graduate education.

Bronk was chairman of the National Research Council of the National Academy of Sciences from 1946 to 1950, and in 1950 he became president of the Academy. It was also in 1950 that the National Science Foundation was formed, and Bronk became chairman of the Foundation's National Science Board. Through these leadership positions Bronk was at the center of White House–level discussions for organizing and promoting scientific research in government agencies and the nation's universities. In 1950 President Truman's advisor William Golden met with Bronk to discuss a proposal to establish a science advisor to the president. No science advisor was appointed then, but a Science Advisory Committee, Office of Defense Mobilization, was formed with Bronk as a member.

As president of the National Academy of Sciences, Bronk was a leader in organizing the International Geophysical Year in 1957 and 1958. Several years in planning, this was a coordinated international effort to study the earth and its cosmic environment, and it included the development of rocket-launched satellites.

On October 4, 1957, the Soviet Union stunned project leaders with the announcement that it had put the first Sputnik satellite into orbit, a breakthrough whose secret development violated agreements for collaboration during the International Geophysical Year. President Eisenhower called Bronk to the White House for advice on his public response to Sputnik. "We decided that his remarks to the press should begin: 'We

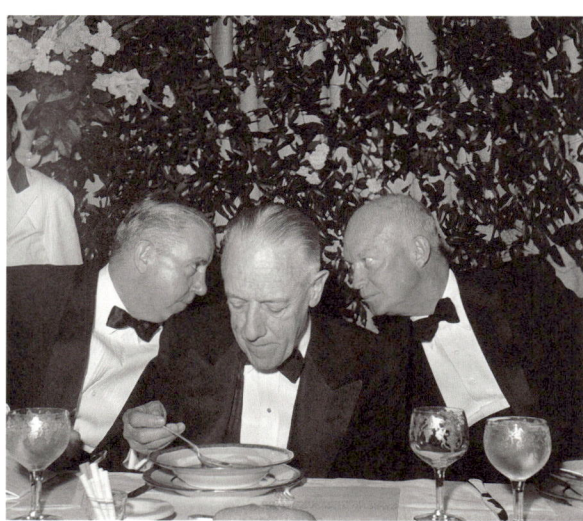

In May 1959 Detlev Bronk (center) dined with President Dwight Eisenhower (right) and James R. Killian, the president's special assistant for science and technology.

At the centennial convocation of the National Academy of Sciences in 1963, from left: Jerome B. Weisner, science advisor to the president; President John F. Kennedy; Detlev Bronk, president of The Rockefeller University; Frederick Seitz, president of the Academy. Seitz later became president of The Rockefeller University and has served as advisor to many government agencies.

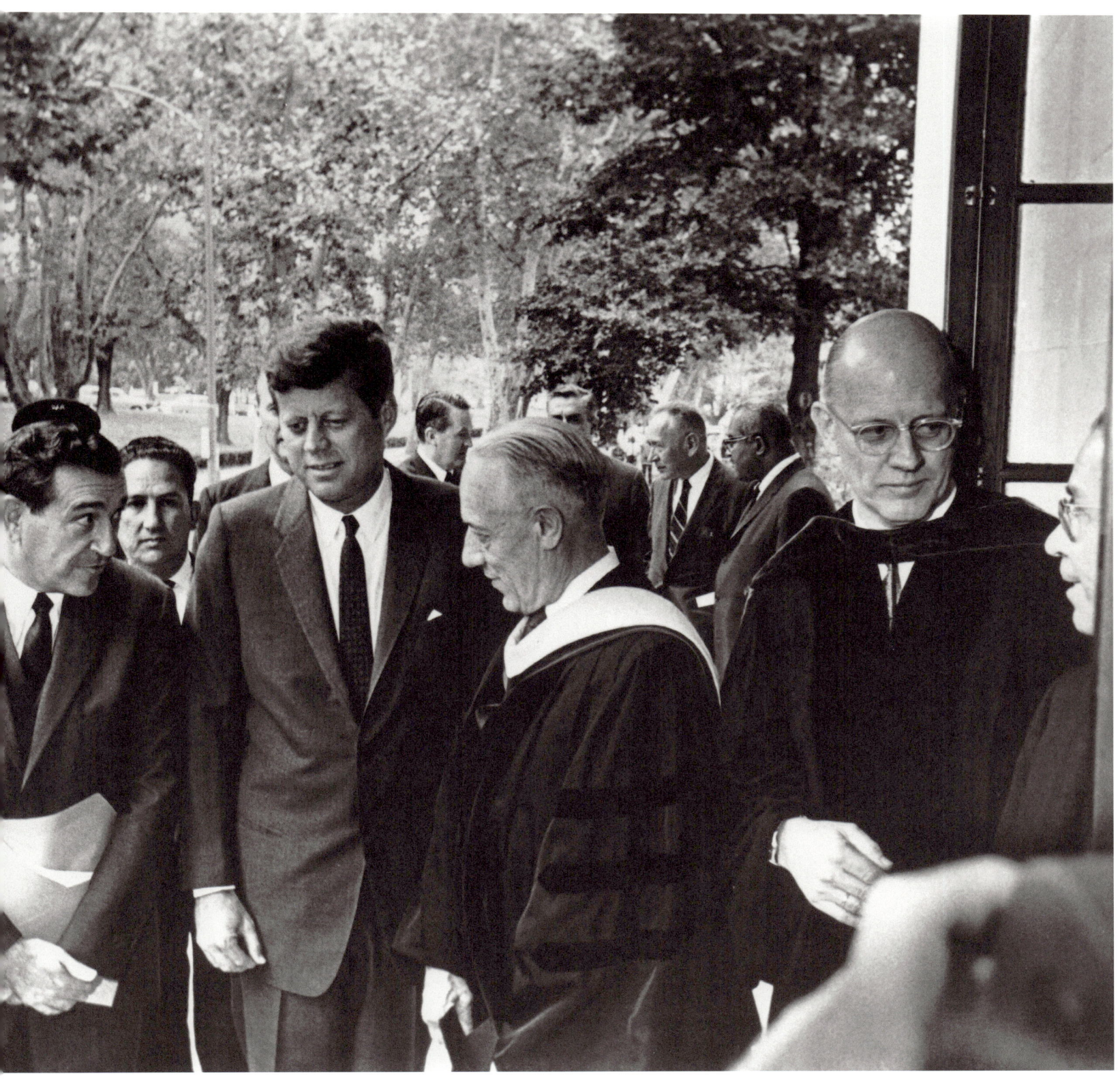

congratulate Russian scientists upon having put their satellite into orbit,'" Bronk recalled, a statement in keeping with Eisenhower's earlier pledge that research during the Geophysical Year should demonstrate the ability of peoples of all nations to work together harmoniously for the common good.

Eisenhower asked Bronk and others for further advice on ensuring the vigor of American science. They agreed that the moment had arrived to appoint a full-time science advisor to the president. Within a few months Eisenhower chose James R. Killian, president of the Massachusetts Institute of Technology, as his special assistant for science and technology. Bronk became a member of the President's Science Advisory Committee, which supported Killian, and chairman of its Panel on International Science, posts he held until 1963.

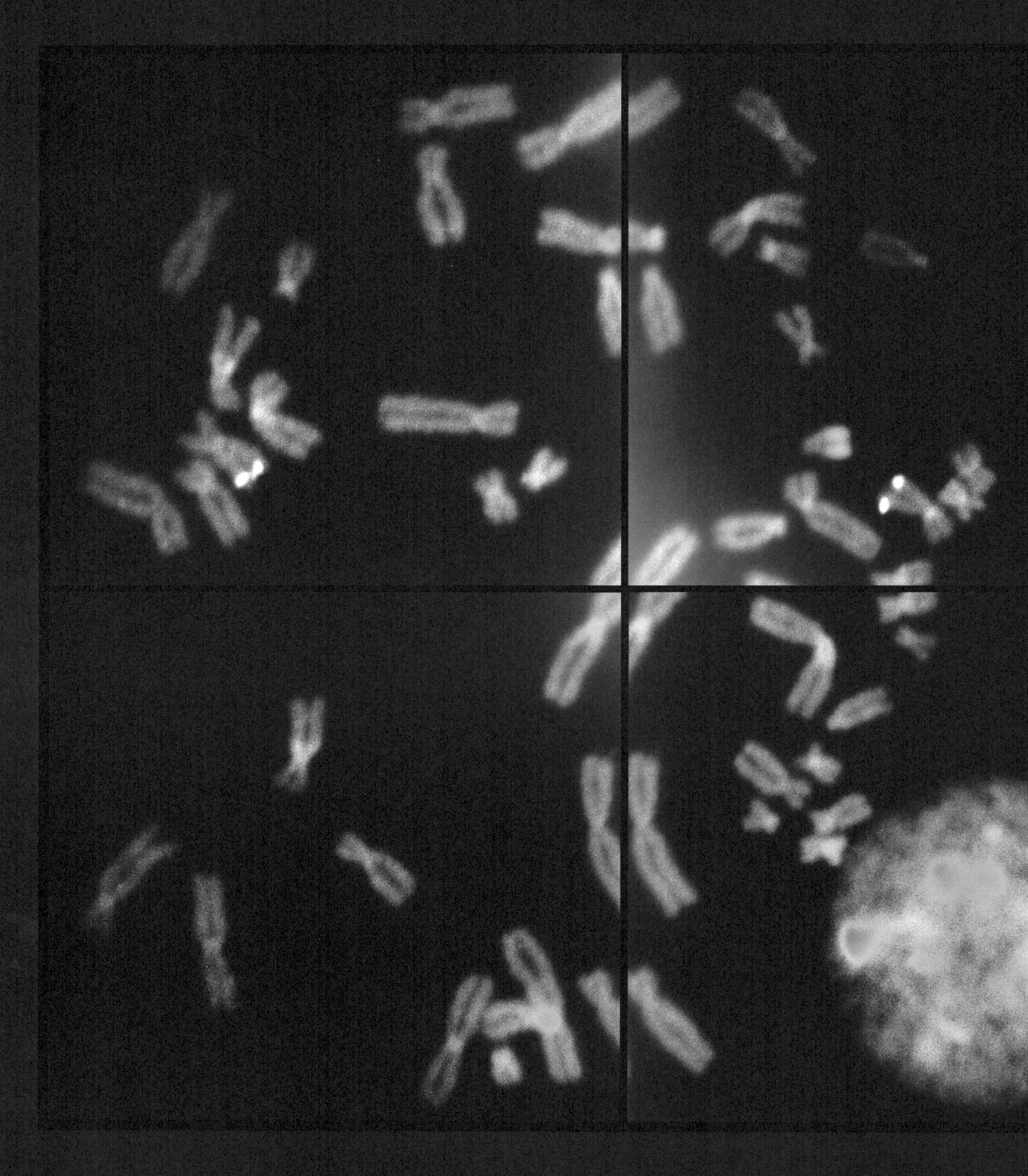

BIOLOGY, CHEMISTRY, AND PHYSICS IN THE AGE OF THE GENE

Part 4: Into the Future

Human chromosomes from two cell nuclei. The chromosomes have been tagged with a fluorescent marker for a tumor suppressor gene.

As The Rockefeller University looks forward to its second century, the vision of its founders remains intact. Ideas that were bold 100 years ago proved to be farsighted, and remain so today. The Rockefeller Institute for Medical Research started as an experiment based on Frederick Gates' hypothesis, supported by John D. Rockefeller, that providing researchers with the resources for "uninterrupted study and investigation" would yield both new knowledge and improved disease treatments.

Simon Flexner set the parameters for this experiment, calculated to harness the new opportunities for medical research that he observed in his own experience as a laboratory scientist. Flexner believed that the collective wealth of science—chemistry and physics as well as biology—should be applied to understanding disease, and that new insights would be gained by seeking out the most original thinkers and giving them resources to do their work. Most important was the freedom to seek new knowledge without looking ahead to its possible application and without the bureaucratic constraints of university departments. The Institute's founders believed that basic research, in the long term, would produce benefits for humankind.

The Rockefeller experiment proved to be productive. Measured in terms of prestigious awards to its faculty—20 Nobel Prizes, 16 Albert Lasker Awards, 5 MacArthur Foundation "genius" awards, and 11 National Medals of Science—it has been a stunning success over the course of a century. The Rockefeller experiment, like any good experiment, was also highly successful when replicated. The Rockefeller laboratories and Hospital served as important models for university research efforts and clinical research centers established in the 20th century.

Rockefeller's ability to thrive amid the many changes of the past 100 years demonstrates the robust nature of the founders' vision. The University has grown from its modest beginnings as a grant-giving institute to 75 laboratories with 140 graduate students and a scientific and administrative staff of 1,800, housed in 19 buildings on a 15-acre campus. The Institute's budget for 1902 was $20,000 and the year ended with a $1,163 surplus. By the end of the century, annual expenditures were nearly $150 million. With physical growth has come expansion in the number of areas of research in the laboratories. Early on, the Institute defined medical research to include the physical sciences, and physicists and mathematicians joined the faculty as Detlev Bronk transformed the Institute into a University. Research today falls into six loosely defined areas: biochemistry, structural biology, and chemistry; molecular, cell,

Harnessing Information

With so many genes directing so many proteins in cells, how do researchers home in on the ones related to specific diseases? In the last decade, as the amount of information about DNA sequences has multiplied, the field of bioinformatics has developed to help answer this question. At Rockefeller, Terry Gaasterland creates computer programs that analyze large databases of genetic information. Andrej Šali is a biophysicist who also takes a computational approach to biology, developing a computer program that predicts the three-dimensional structure of proteins from the information provided by DNA. Both Gaasterland and Šali collaborate with many other researchers at Rockefeller.

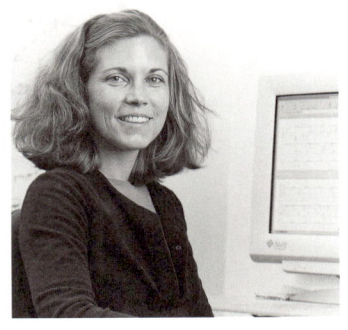

Terry Gaasterland heads the laboratory of computational genomics.

and developmental biology; immunology, virology, and microbiology; medical sciences and human genetics; neuroscience; and physics and mathematical biology. In addition, seven research centers facilitate collaborations without imposing bureaucracy.

Despite this growth Rockefeller remains an intimate institution by the standards of research universities. Following a decades-old tradition, staff and students gather for tea and a scientific lecture on Friday afternoons. President Levine extends his hospitality to the community, hosting dinners at his house with smaller groups of faculty, students, and other guests. Although new research buildings rise high above the south end of the campus, the 66th Street gate looks much the same as when it was erected in 1915. The verdant campus, a retreat from the bustle and noise of the surrounding city, provides a serene environment that sustains intense intellectual endeavor. The first step through the gates leading up the tree-lined hill to Founder's Hall begins a walk that has been familiar to scientists for a century.

The University also remains steadfast in its commitment to expanding the boundaries of knowledge. Over the course of a century education has become an increasingly important component of Rockefeller's mission. The graduate program remains unique in its emphasis on learning through mentoring and hands-on research rather than class work. To prepare for the interdisciplinary nature of science today, students undergo rigorous scientific cross-training, rotating through different laboratories until they have acquired the necessary skills and knowledge to embark on an original project. For example, one student is pursuing research that spans mass spectroscopy, synthetic protein chemistry, and molecular biology. Many others list two faculty members as their thesis advisors. Acting on the conviction that the scientific leaders of tomorrow must be broadly educated, the University provides students with opportunities to hear lectures on literature, the fine arts, and music, and to enjoy concerts in Caspary Auditorium. The University's location also gives students easy access to the cultural resources of New York City.

In addition, The Rockefeller University's education efforts include a summer research program for undergraduates, events and research programs for high school students and their teachers, presentations for journalists, and lectures for the general public. The University continually seeks ways to enrich the intellectual life of diverse communities and to broaden public understanding of science.

Since the University's founding, its Upper East Side neighborhood has developed in ways that facilitate collaboration with New York City's scientific community. Rockefeller shares the corner of 68th Street and York Avenue with Weill Medical College of Cornell University at New York–Presbyterian Hospital and the Memorial Sloan-Kettering Cancer Center. This tri-institutional scientific community shares both scientific seminars and cultural events. The many other outstanding research centers in the New York metropolitan area provide opportunities for further institutional collaborations. For example, Rockefeller is working with other universities and hospitals to gain access to large populations of patients for studies of the genetic components of diseases such as diabetes, schizophrenia, and cancer, to share complex laboratory equipment, and to enhance undergraduate educational programs.

The Nobel Prize, 1999

Cell biologist Günter Blobel was awarded the 1999 Nobel Prize in Physiology or Medicine for the discovery that "proteins have intrinsic signals that govern their transport and localization in the cell." Blobel came to Rockefeller in 1967, joining the laboratory of pioneering cell biologists George Palade and Philip Siekevitz. He is also an investigator at the Howard Hughes Medical Institute.

Interdisciplinary Science

At Rockefeller today, much scientific work focuses on gaining a detailed understanding of how genes work at the level of individual molecules. Advances in both basic biology and medicine depend on understanding how the DNA code is regulated so as to manufacture proteins in cells, and how those proteins—hormones, chemical messengers, antibodies, ion channels, and enzymes, for example—function.

"It is clear that science has entered an era dominated by the study of genes," says president Arnold Levine. The completion of the human genome project is giving scientists a giant boost in this endeavor, providing them with the letter-by-letter instructions encoded in DNA.

The University has always encouraged scientific collaborations across disciplinary boundaries, and studying genes and their proteins today requires chemists, physicists, and biologists to work together in ways that Simon Flexner could not have imagined. Physicists, for example, are lending their expertise to interpreting the information encoded in DNA. From their perspective this information is encoded much like the language of a computer program, so the tools of information technology can be applied to analyzing and manipulating it. The string of letters that describes a given stretch of DNA can be organized into something analogous to words, sentences,

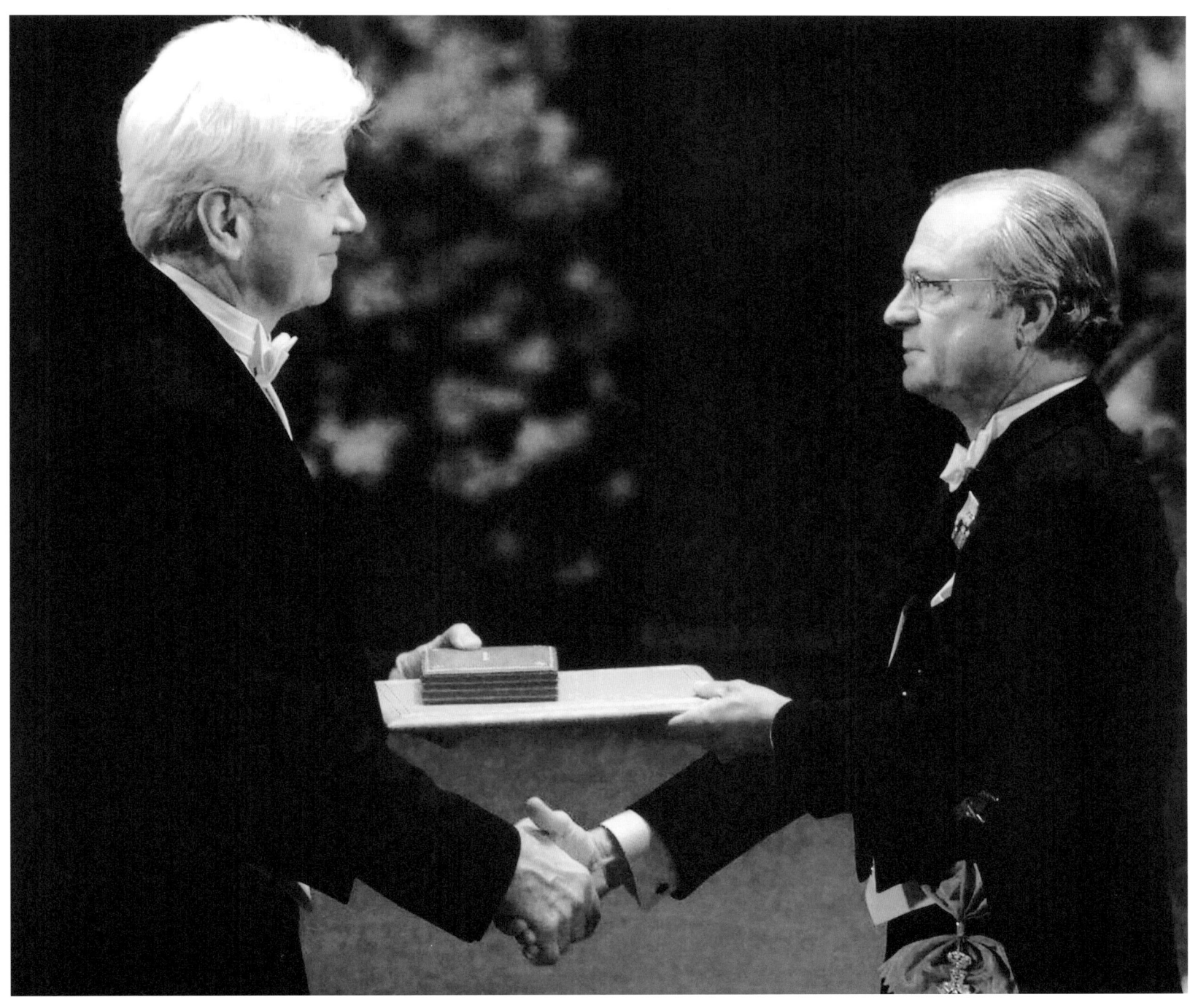

Günter Blobel (left) accepting his Nobel Prize from the king of Sweden.

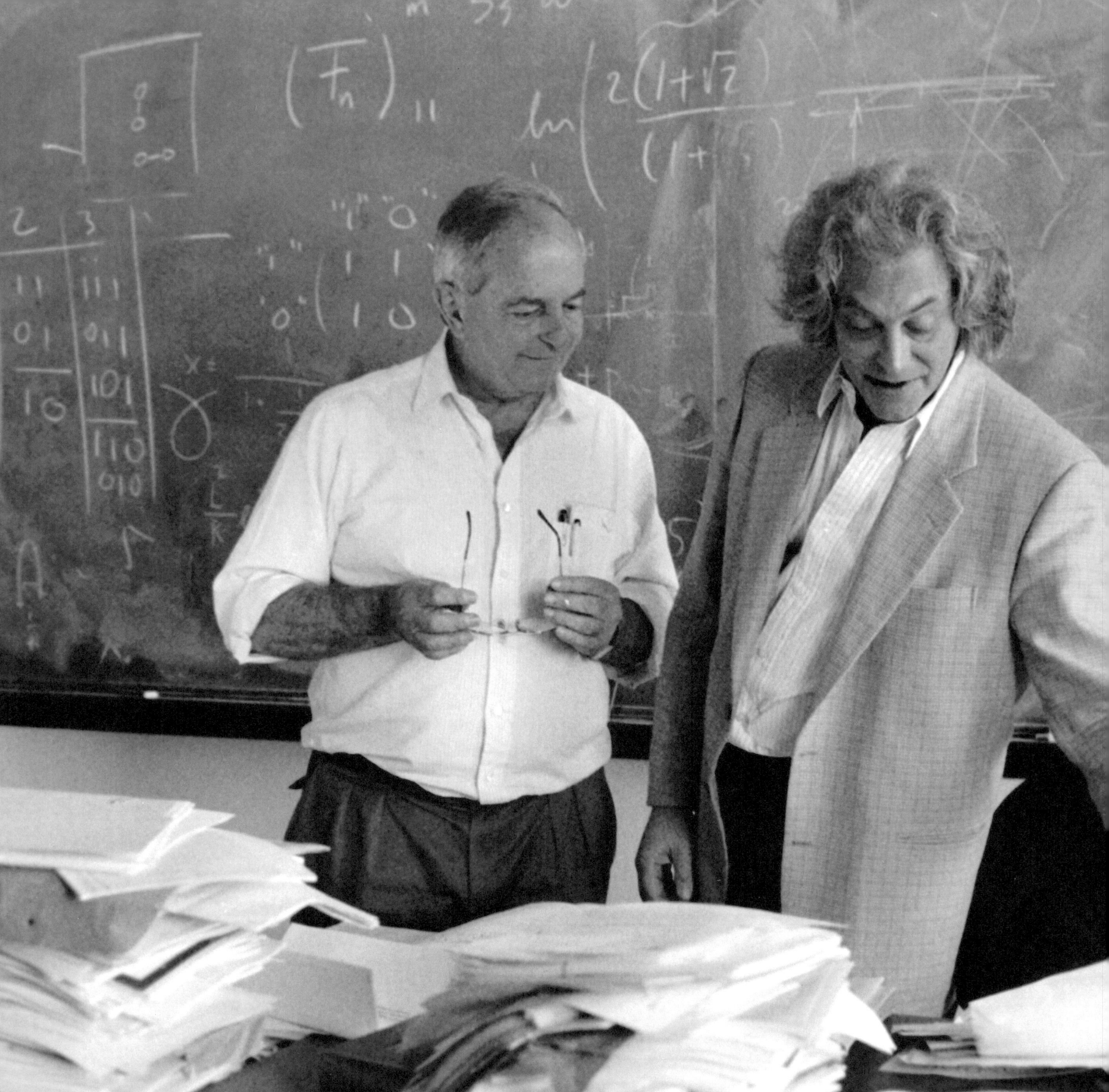

and books. "Having that information, we can start to think of a language of life," says physicist Albert Libchaber. "This won't be done in a wet lab, it will be done with computers. Mathematicians and physicists are working together to get that grammar."

One step toward parsing the DNA language involves creating DNA chips, which are fingernail-sized arrays containing snippets of known genes. With these, researchers can test which genes in a DNA sample are "turned on"—expressed as messenger RNA in a cell. Just as computer chips make it possible to store and manipulate digital information, DNA chips allow scientists to analyze and compare vast amounts of genetic information. With DNA chips, for example, Libchaber and his colleagues can "tell which sentences in the DNA book the cell is using," and compare normal and cancerous cells. Such new technologies are leading to better ways of diagnosing disease.

Chemists and biologists also are collaborating in new ways to understand the details of how proteins function in cells. "Cell biology," Levine says, "a field that was born at Rockefeller more than 50 years ago, is undergoing a profound transformation thanks to the contributions of chemists."

Cell biologist and 1999 Nobel laureate Günter Blobel describes these interdisciplinary collaborations as "a tremendously rich soup" in which each ingredient contributes to the quality of understanding. Biochemistry and cell biology focus on the functions of proteins, he says, and structural biology "looks at high-resolution structures of the proteins. There is also chemistry to modify the structure of the proteins." Computational biologists, he adds, focus on the gene sequences for particular proteins, comparing the sequences to find clues to how the proteins function.

Blobel's award-winning work has involved many such collaborations, particularly among cell biology, biochemistry, and structural biology. His research predicted and revealed the existence of a "ZIP code" system in the cell, by which newly made proteins are directed to specific addresses. Making proteins and shipping them to appropriate destinations, such as the cell's internal organelles, is a vital activity in cells. Blobel's work showed that each newly made protein has an organelle-specific address, a stretch of the protein referred to as a signal sequence that is recognized by an organelle's surface. His laboratory's findings have an immediate bearing on many diseases, including cystic fibrosis, Alzheimer's disease, and AIDS.

Physicists Albert Libchaber (left) and Mitchell J. Feigenbaum pioneered experimental and mathematical approaches to nonlinear dynamics, or chaos theory.

As a continuation of the work of the founders of cell biology, Blobel's achievements are deeply rooted in the University's past. Rockefeller's history both informs and inspires the research of today. The work of many laboratories builds on long intellectual lineages not only in cell biology, but also in microbiology, immunology, and protein chemistry. Other areas that were strengths in Rockefeller's past, such as cancer biology and virology, are now receiving renewed support.

When Rockefeller was founded infectious diseases constituted the most important threat to health. With the discovery of antibiotics in the mid-20th century, it seemed possible to conquer many of these diseases, or at least hold them in check. However, at the turn of the 21st century a resurgence in infectious diseases has made research into their underlying causes a priority again, and Rockefeller is building a team of scientists with complementary expertise in this area. Fighting antibiotic-resistant bacteria and viruses such as HIV and hepatitis C requires the resources of microbiology, genetics, and immunology as well as structural biology and chemistry. Joining forces across these disciplines, Rockefeller scientists are identifying the molecular mechanisms that cause these diseases and designing new therapies to treat them.

Tuberculosis is a particularly persistent infection; it was a dangerous disease that concerned Rockefeller researchers at the beginning of the century and, although suppressed for many years, it has recently reemerged as a threat to public health. Tuberculosis is also persistent in infected individuals, eluding both antibiotics and the body's immune defenses and allowing victims to live for years while unknowingly spreading the infection to others. Today tuberculosis accounts for 3 million deaths each year worldwide. John McKinney is taking a genetic approach to finding the tuberculosis bacterium's molecular vulnerabilities. "A major aim of these studies is to identify molecular targets for developing new and more effective anti-tuberculosis therapies," he says.

Diverse approaches to the challenge of bacteria that resist treatment with antibiotics are being developed in several Rockefeller laboratories. Cell biologist Alexander Tomasz is tracking the spread of antibiotic-resistant bacteria and the cellular changes that enable them to survive treatment with today's drugs. For some bacteria, antibiotic resistance is tied to a particular enzyme. When such a molecule is pinpointed, scientists can take steps to impede its activity in a cell. Structural biologists approach this problem by determining the three-dimensional form of a molecule. Knowing this, they can attempt to fit smaller molecules into pockets in the structure to block its

Alzheimer's Evidence

In Alzheimer's disease, deposits of proteins build up in the brain. These protein plaques, as they are called, appear in all cases of Alzheimer's, although scientists do not yet fully understand their role in the disease. Neuroscientist Paul Greengard has found that treating animal and human nerve cells with the sex hormones estrogen and testosterone greatly reduces the accumulation of protein plaques. The brain is made up of nerve cells, so this discovery provides the first molecular and cellular evidence of why estrogen replacement therapy offers postmenopausal women some protection against Alzheimer's, and suggests that testosterone supplementation may protect against Alzheimer's in elderly men.

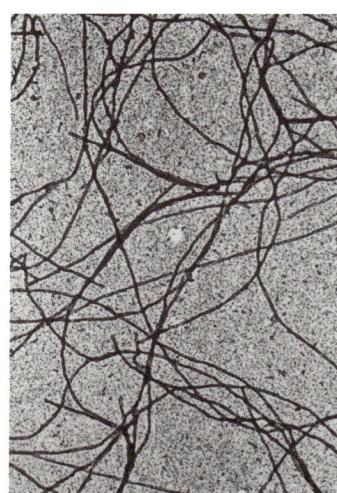

Protein plaques—tangled masses of protein filaments—are associated with Alzheimer's disease.

function. Biophysicist Stephen Burley and his colleagues have determined the three-dimensional structure of an enzyme responsible for resistance of certain bacteria to the antibiotic gentamicin. The enzyme's structure resembles a right hand cupped as though wrapped around a cylinder. The cavity produced by the cupped hand presents a possible target for drugs aimed at thwarting antibiotic resistance.

Chemists can tailor-make new molecules, designing compounds that are aimed at such targets. One molecule developed by synthetic chemist Tom Muir turns off virulence in staphylococcus bacteria. This and other bacteria become more aggressively infectious when they reach a certain density of growth, so Muir and his colleagues designed a molecule that inhibits this phenomenon. They are modifying this molecule, ultimately to be tried as a potential treatment in people as an alternative to antibiotics.

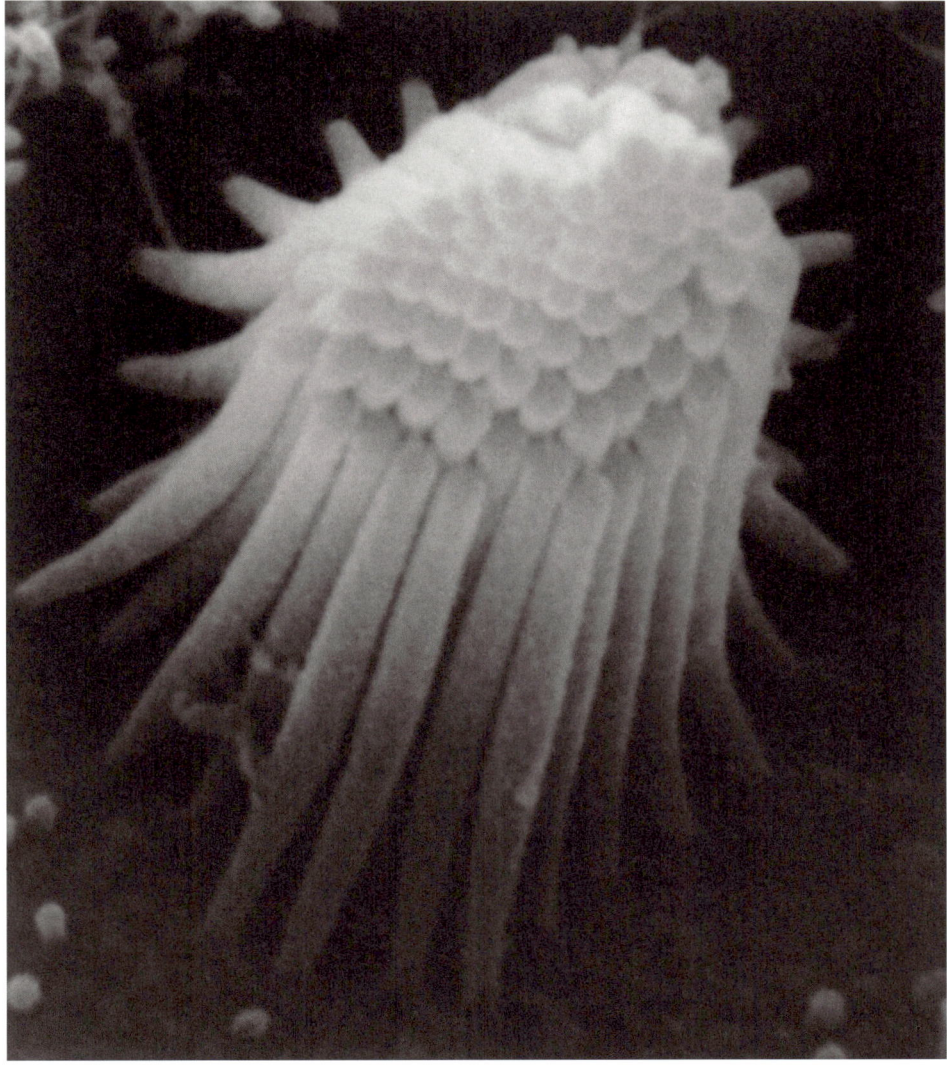

A hair cell in the ear.

Amplifiers in the Ear

Hearing depends on cellular receptors in the ear relaying sound signals to the brain. Neuroscientist A. James Hudspeth has found that these cells, known as hair cells, can amplify sound and augment the sensitivity of hearing. The "hairs" seen in the photograph protrude from a single cell.

The problems of controlling infectious diseases are the focus not only of biologists and chemists at Rockefeller, but also of mathematicians such as Joel Cohen. Among other things, Cohen studies the patterns and conditions of transmission of Chagas' disease, an insect-borne infection that afflicts millions of people in Latin America. His laboratory is developing a mathematical model of how transmission occurs, a project that will lead to an understanding of how people can lower their risk of infection.

Much of the research on infectious diseases is done at Rockefeller's Hospital, which remains as central to the University's future as it was to the past. The Hospital today is home to studies of human genetics, immunology, cancer biology, and many other areas of medical science. Inside the same building where clinical research was pioneered, the link between basic research and clinical investigation remains as strong as ever.

At the Rockefeller Hospital the multidrug AIDS "cocktail" was tested, which dramatically reduces virus levels in certain patients. The Aaron Diamond AIDS Research Center—the world's largest private HIV/AIDS research institute—has been affiliated with the University since 1996. That year David Ho, the Aaron Diamond Center's founding director, was appointed to The Rockefeller University faculty. Work at the Aaron Diamond Center on the molecular dynamics of HIV infection led to the development of this drug regimen.

The Next 100 Years

A century after its founding, Rockefeller's institutional structure of independent laboratories remains unique and continues to make possible groundbreaking science. A part of the University's success can be attributed to the flexibility of the structure, a capacity for change that Simon Flexner built into his organization of the original Institute.

"The direction of scientific investigation changes from decade to decade," wrote Flexner, "and often with startling and unforeseen suddenness." By choosing not to staff the Institute like a well-rounded university department, Flexner freed himself to take risks and to hire scientists who were leading medical research in new directions. "It is…an institution in which opportunism, in the best sense of the word, plays a determining role," he wrote.

Young Talent

Every year 15 college undergraduates and 50 high school students spend their summer vacation at Rockefeller getting hands-on experience in laboratory research. Faculty mentoring and science immersion pay off: about 10 percent of the high school students become Intel Science Talent Search semifinalists, and many go on to be finalists and winners. The University also sponsors summer programs for high school teachers.

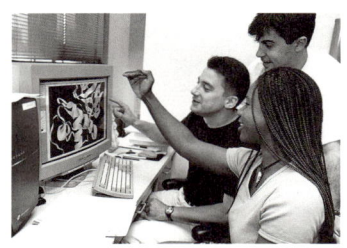

Rockefeller's Marcus Albertini and Robby Allario work with Karen McFarlane, an undergraduate at the City University of New York, in the laboratory of Günter Blobel.

The built-in flexibility of the institution provides opportunities to expand the intellectual life of the University by hiring researchers in new fields as particular scientific problems become urgent and allowing current faculty to change research focus. The hepatitis C virus, for example, was not isolated or identified a decade ago, but today we know it has infected 4 million people in the United States and causes as many as 10,000 deaths annually. To address this problem, Charles Rice joined the faculty to lead an interdisciplinary team investigating the basic biology of the virus, its clinical manifestations in patients, and the development of new treatments. The Center for the Study of Hepatitis C, which Rice heads, was established jointly among Rockefeller, New York–Presbyterian Hospital, and Weill Medical College of Cornell University, taking advantage of the scientific resources of the University's 68th Street neighborhood.

At the beginning of Rockefeller's second century, there is remarkable continuity with the past. For 100 years the University has remained committed to fostering the most creative approaches to scientific problems. John D. Rockefeller's founding pledge took a far-reaching view of the future, and that philosophy has sustained long-term basic research projects for decades. Through the century and through the generations the Rockefeller family members, especially John D. Rockefeller Jr. and David Rockefeller, have affirmed and extended their pioneering support for research through their involvement in the University's administration as well as their philanthropy. The University can justly boast of a century of accomplishments that have in large part charted the course of biomedical science.

The clear vision of the future of science that Rockefeller's founders articulated—medical research based on the contributions of the physical sciences as well as biology—remains fresh and productive today as chemistry and physics become increasingly important to the study of biology. At the beginning of the 21st century, The Rockefeller University seeks to provide future generations with science that benefits all.

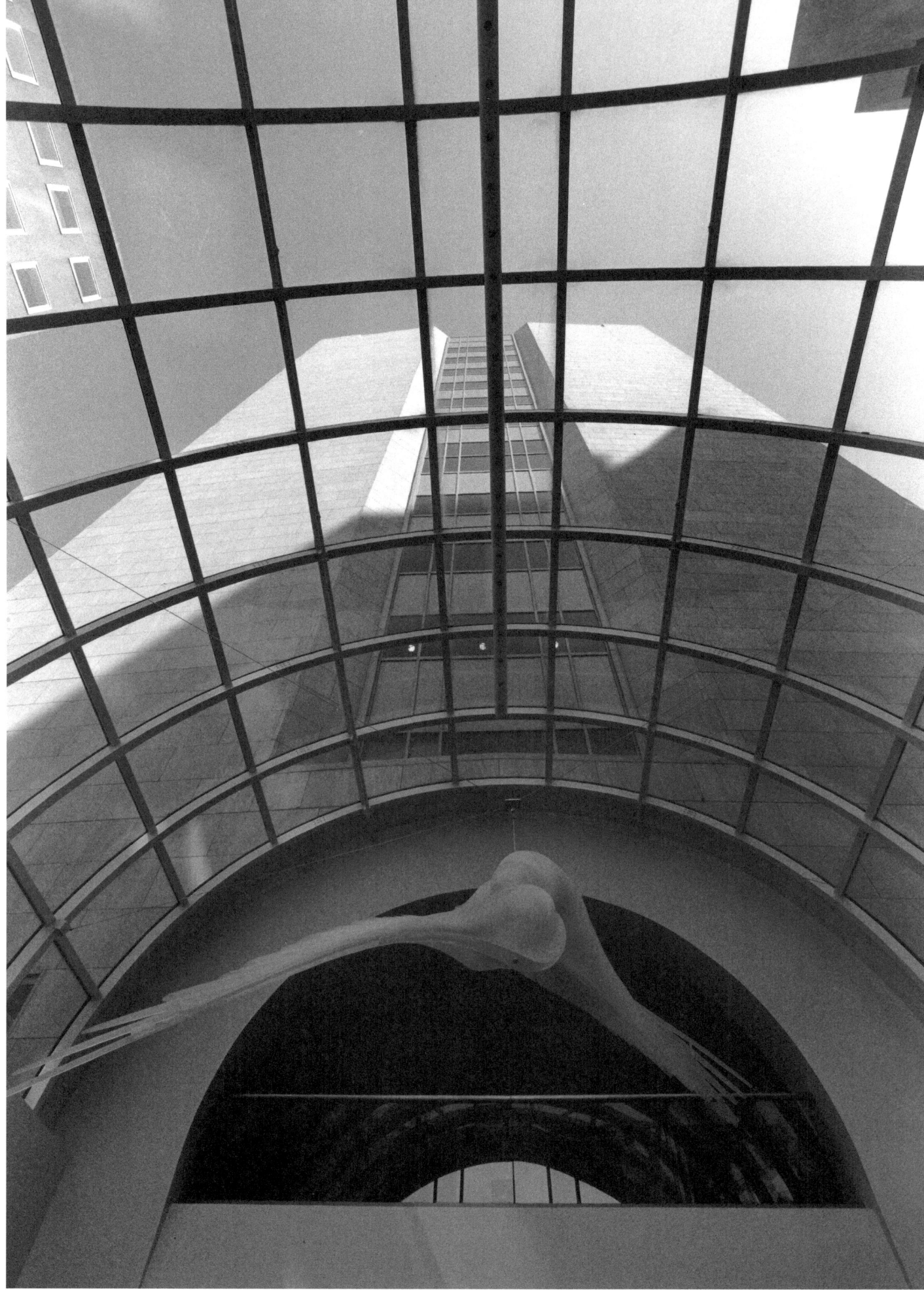

The John D. Rockefeller Jr. and David Rockefeller Research Building.

BIOLOGY, CHEMISTRY, AND PHYSICS IN THE AGE OF THE GENE

A Closer Look: Into the Future

Gene-Hunting in the South Pacific 128

A Graduate's Tribute 130

Cancer Fundamentals 133

Charging Up Immune Defenses 134

The Body Electric 136

Chromosomal End Game 139

The Chemistry of Life 140

Gene-Hunting in the South Pacific

Obesity, heart disease, and diabetes are disorders caused in part by genetic predisposition. The three disorders are related through obesity—obese people are more likely than others to suffer from heart problems and diabetes. However, unlike other diseases that may be caused by a single gene, this trio of ailments results from the interplay of many genes in combination with environmental influences and lifestyle.

The likelihood of finding genes linked to obesity, heart disease, and diabetes might seem hopelessly small, but scientists at Rockefeller University's Starr Center for Human Genetics have a research plan that increases their odds. They are studying the DNA, medical histories, and family trees of a group of people whose genes are remarkably similar and who suffer disproportionately from these disorders.

These people live on the island of Kosrae, in Micronesia. Since the island became a U.S. protectorate after World War II its population has grown from about 300 to more than 8,000. This expansion is the result of Kosraeans having large families, as few people from elsewhere have settled on the island. At the same time, with the introduction of fatty Western foods such as tinned meat and ice cream, more than half the adults on Kosrae have become obese, and one in eight suffers from adult-onset, or Type 2, diabetes.

The studies are a collaboration with the Kosrae Department of Health and Rockefeller scientists Jeffrey Friedman, director of the Starr Center, who isolated the gene *obese* and the protein leptin, which influence obesity; Jan Breslow, who has found a gene that predisposes people to heart disease; and Markus Stoffel, who studies diabetes in patients at the Rockefeller Hospital. Maria Karayiorgou, another Starr Center researcher, collaborates by using the Kosrae data to search for genes that contribute to psychiatric illnesses such as schizophrenia and obsessive-compulsive disorder.

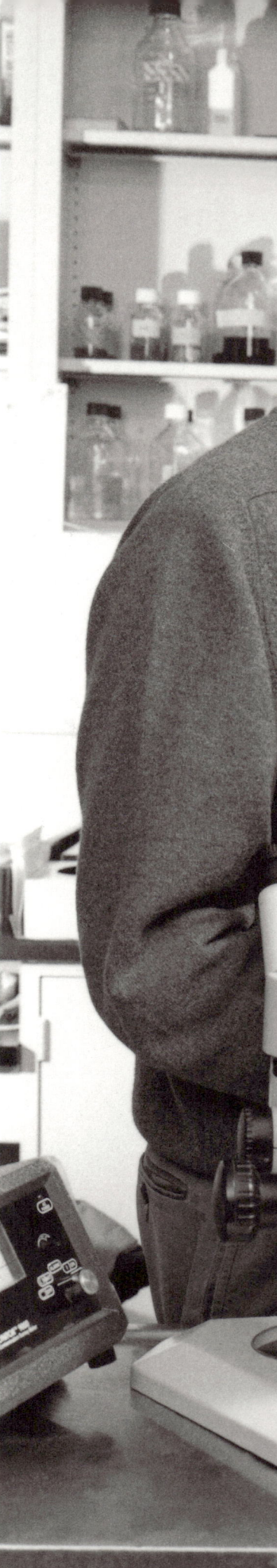

Markus Stoffel (left) with post-doctoral fellow Maria Angeles Navas and biomedical fellow David Shih in the laboratory of metabolic diseases.

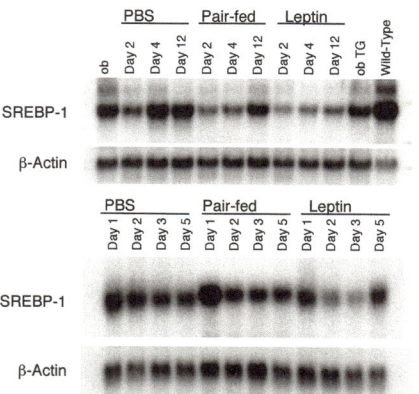

Analyses of the effects of the protein leptin, which influences obesity, on production of another protein, called SREBP-1, from research in the laboratory of Jeffrey Friedman.

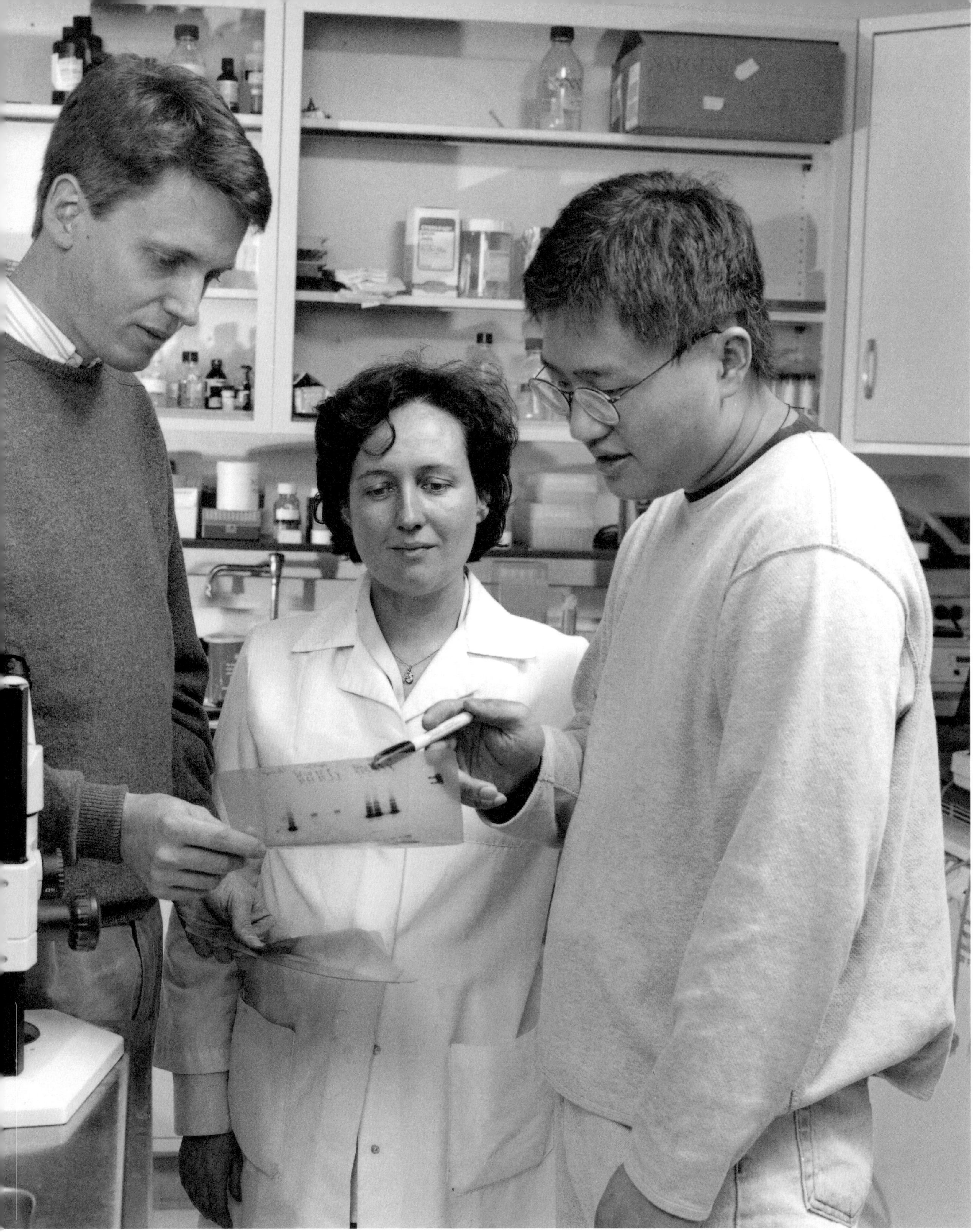

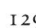

A Graduate's Tribute

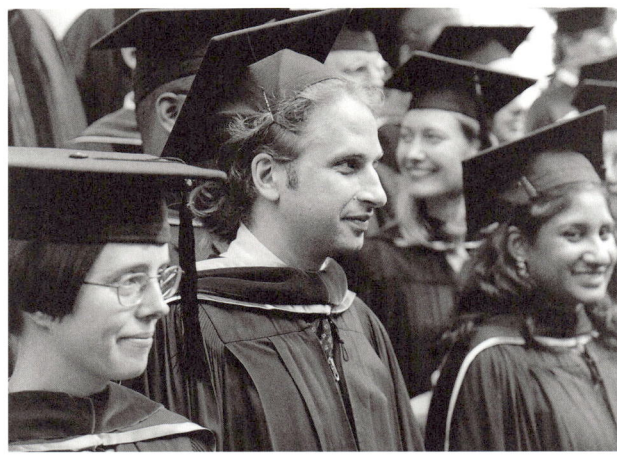

Matthew Albert, a 1999 Rockefeller graduate, delivered the speech excerpted below at his Convocation. Albert also received the 1999 Council of Graduate Schools/ University Microfilms International Distinguished Dissertation Award.

"When I first introduce visitors or colleagues to Rockefeller, I usually begin at the Faculty and Students Club. This might seem like an odd place to start,...but in so many ways, the club reflects the Rockefeller community. Still decorated as I imagine it was in the 1950s, with a dusty model of the structure of DNA in the corner, it is a place of no pretense. There is a complete lack of protocol and hierarchy, offering a chance for students and faculty to interact in a relaxed, open and meaningful way. It's not President Levine, Dean Cross or Dr. de Lange. It's Arnie, George and Titia.

"It is this attitude that pervades campus life, as no one here hides behind titles nor even the walls of individual academic departments. Scientific discovery does not respect the boundaries of an Immunology or a Cellular Biology department and the founding members of this community made sure that scientists working at Rockefeller would be free to follow their own paths, not bound by the typical confines of the academy.

"[S]cience is...one of the hardest things we could have chosen, or that has chosen us. Rockefeller students are expected to get right to work. To break a pipette or two along the way, but to get right in there, hands dirty and fast. Classes are offered, but only few are required. We are not spoon-fed as I have experienced at other institutions. No one tells us what to do. And at times that freedom is almost a burden. We feel that we must take advantage of it, do well by it, and work in a way that reflects who we are and how we think.

"At Rockefeller we've had the opportunity to address the ideas burning inside of us. This is our poetry, our art. I watch friends who are artists and writers struggle to figure out how to both survive and do what they love. Almost daily, I am reminded how lucky we are, that where we see poetry is in science, a field where there is much support. Here, that support goes well beyond the financial, and has meant a nurturing community that has given us both the tools and the freedom for responsible scientific explorations."

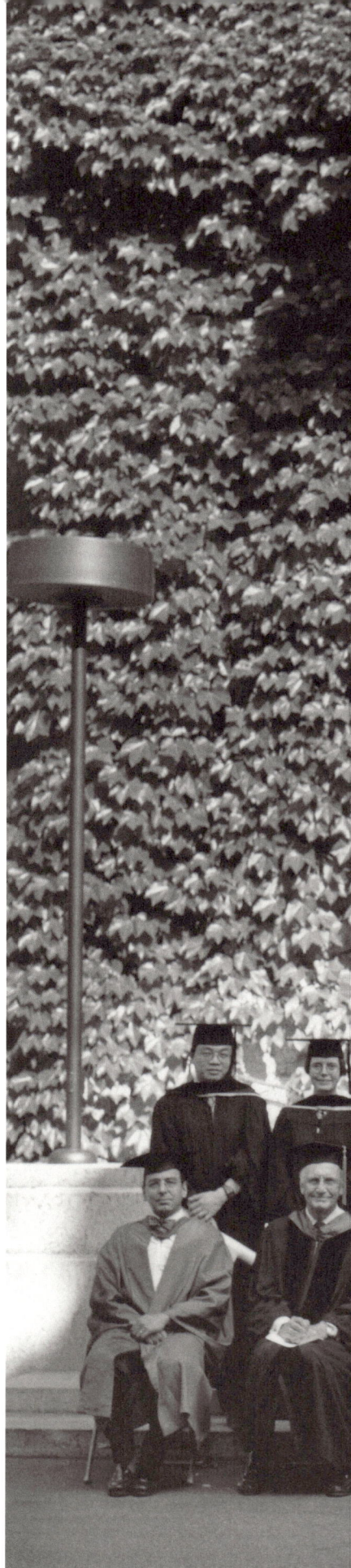

Fiona Doetsch, Matthew Albert, and Rhupal Bhatt (above). Graduates, University faculty, and honorary degree recipients at Convocation in June 1999.

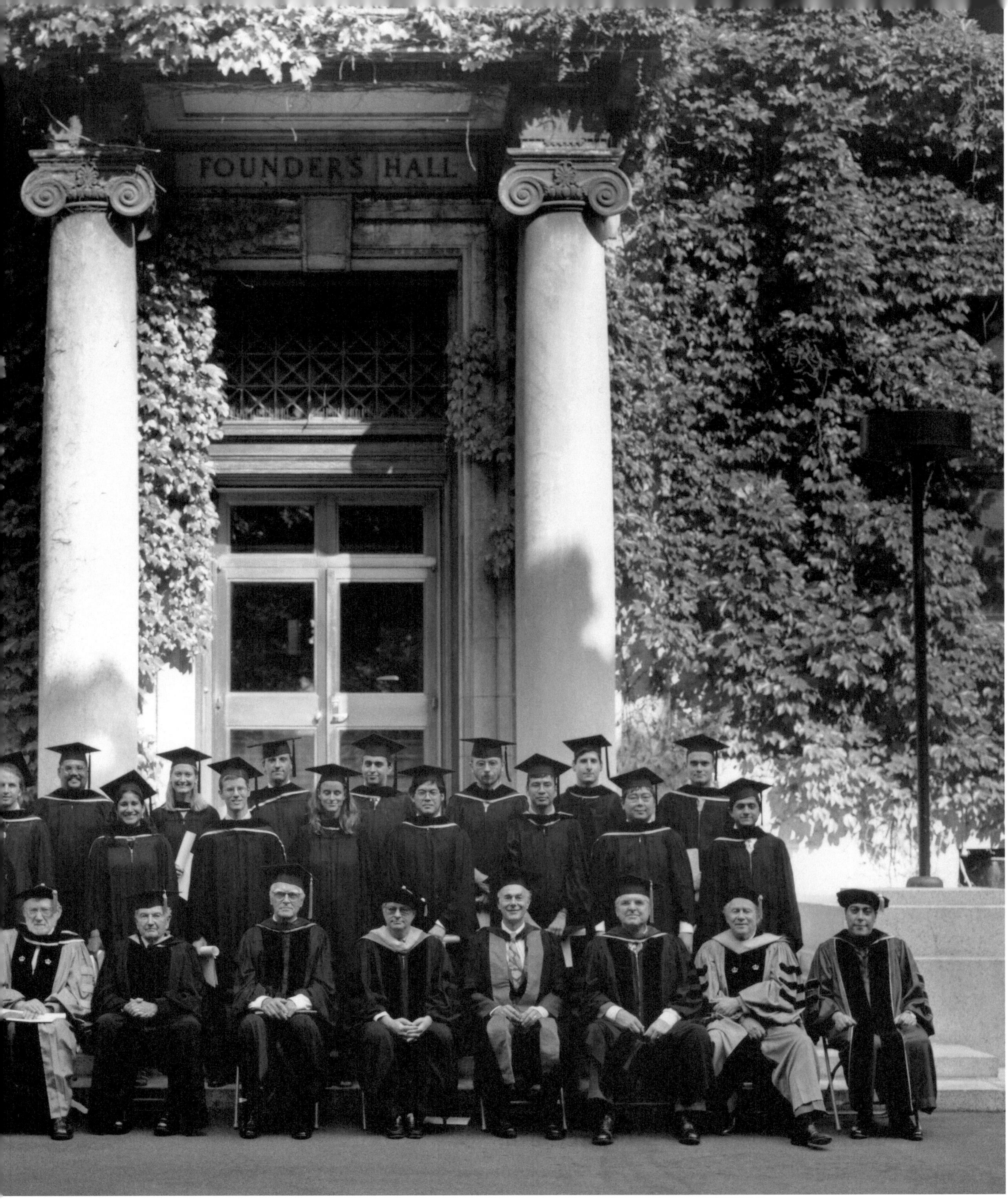

131

Analysis with DNA chip technology shows activation of the p53 tumor suppressor gene.

Cancer Fundamentals

The diseases we lump under the single rubric of cancer—cells reproducing with abandon, often accumulating in tumors—have for decades eluded scientists' efforts to find cures. With advances in understanding cancer at the molecular level, however, researchers are beginning to reap the rewards of long-term investment in studying the disease.

Robert G. Roeder's research delves into one of the most fundamental processes in biology—the way in which genetic information encoded in DNA is converted into protein, a process called gene expression. Roeder's work has focused on the first and most important step in gene expression—making a copy of the DNA. In this process, known as transcription, proteins called gene activators must recognize specific positions on the DNA.

These kinds of proteins were first isolated in Roeder's laboratory in biochemical studies of the molecular mechanism of transcription. The work on transcription is closely tied to the research of other Rockefeller scientists—the tumor suppressor *p53* studied by Arnold Levine, for example, is a gene activator that functions through the transcriptional machinery Roeder has described. Levine discovered the *p53* gene, and his work is leading to ways of improving cancer treatment. In 1999 Roeder and Levine received awards from the General Motors Cancer Research Foundation for their contributions to cancer research.

Research at Rockefeller on another gene-activator protein, called Stat3, has recently yielded groundbreaking results with new-drug potential. James Darnell Jr. and his coworkers discovered in 1999 that the protein Stat3 can cause cancer when it is persistently activated in a cell.

Stat3, which is often activated in breast cancer, stimulates conditions for unrestrained cell growth. Knowing that Stat3 can contribute to the development of tumors, scientists can look for—or try to design—drugs that deactivate the protein.

"We're at that awkward moment in science when we understand how cancer is caused, and we can't do enough to reverse it yet," says Levine, "but now we are prepared for the first time to launch a rational attack to cure this disease."

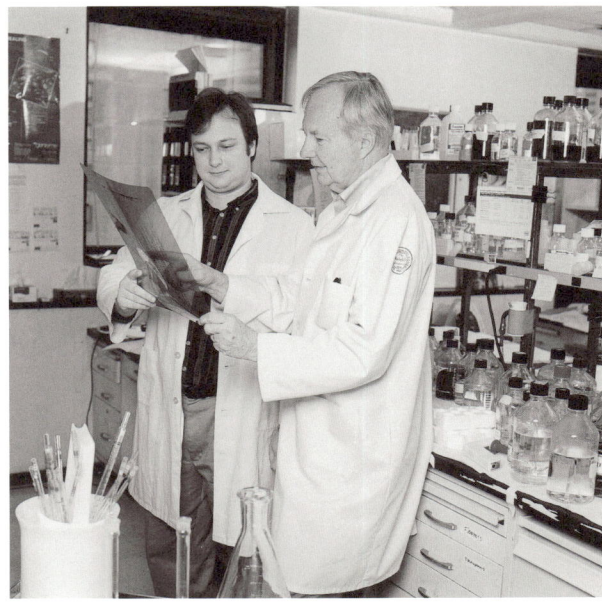

James E. Darnell Jr. (right) studies a protein that can contribute to the development of tumors. With him is graduate fellow Stanislav Mamonov.

Charging Up Immune Defenses

The immune system enlists specialized cells to patrol the body and seek out and destroy infectious microorganisms. Among these, dendritic cells are known as sentinels of the immune system—they set in motion a chain of events that prepare the other cells to fight the invaders. Studies at Rockefeller are showing that dendritic cells also hold a key to unlocking the power of the body's own defense system to heal itself.

Clinical investigator Nina Bhardwaj is using dendritic cells to boost the human immune system to fight infections and cancers. Bhardwaj and her coworkers recently showed that a single injection of dendritic cells, mixed with some of the body's T cells, improves the immune system of healthy people, and this heightened immunity can last for up to three months. She is now extending this technique to treat HIV infections and melanoma.

Neuro-oncologist Robert B. Darnell and coworkers have recently found that for a small percentage of the population the body's immune system mounts an attack against cancer cells, often without the person knowing that a tumor exists. Dendritic cells may offer a route for enhancing this natural tumor immunity in other patients with cancer.

Dendritic cells were discovered at Rockefeller in 1973 by Ralph M. Steinman and the late Zanvil A. Cohn. Steinman continues the work in his laboratory today, focusing on the basic biology of how the cells develop their potency and how they can be used to change the course of disease, especially AIDS. "There are many new insights in reorienting the immune system to deal with viruses like HIV," says Steinman, "maybe not to eliminate them in the way that smallpox and polio were eliminated, but to keep them at an asymptomatic checkmate."

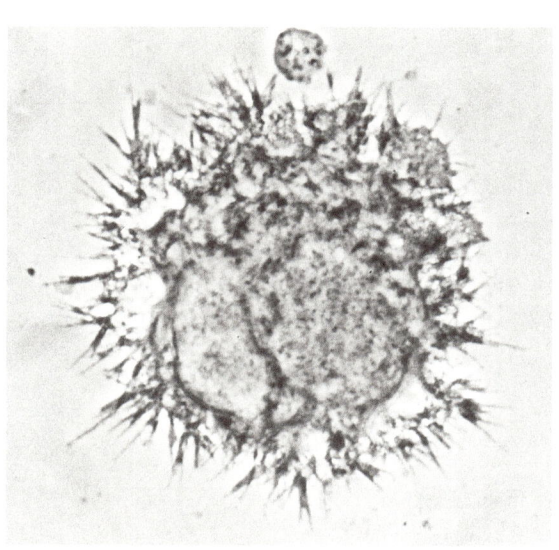

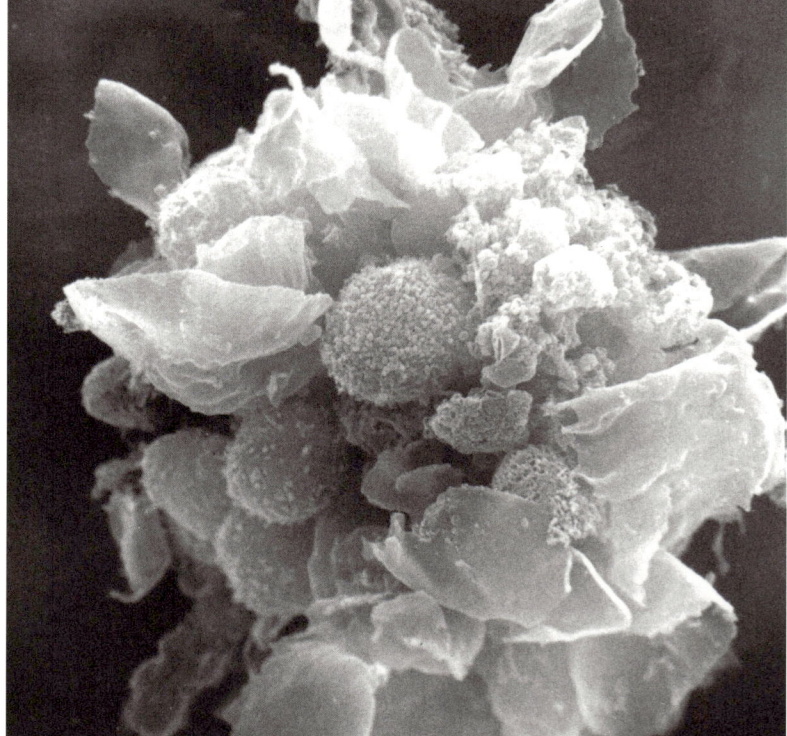

Three views of dendritic cells: isolated from the skin (left), interacting with round T cells (middle), lying inside the skin awaiting the introduction of an infection (right).

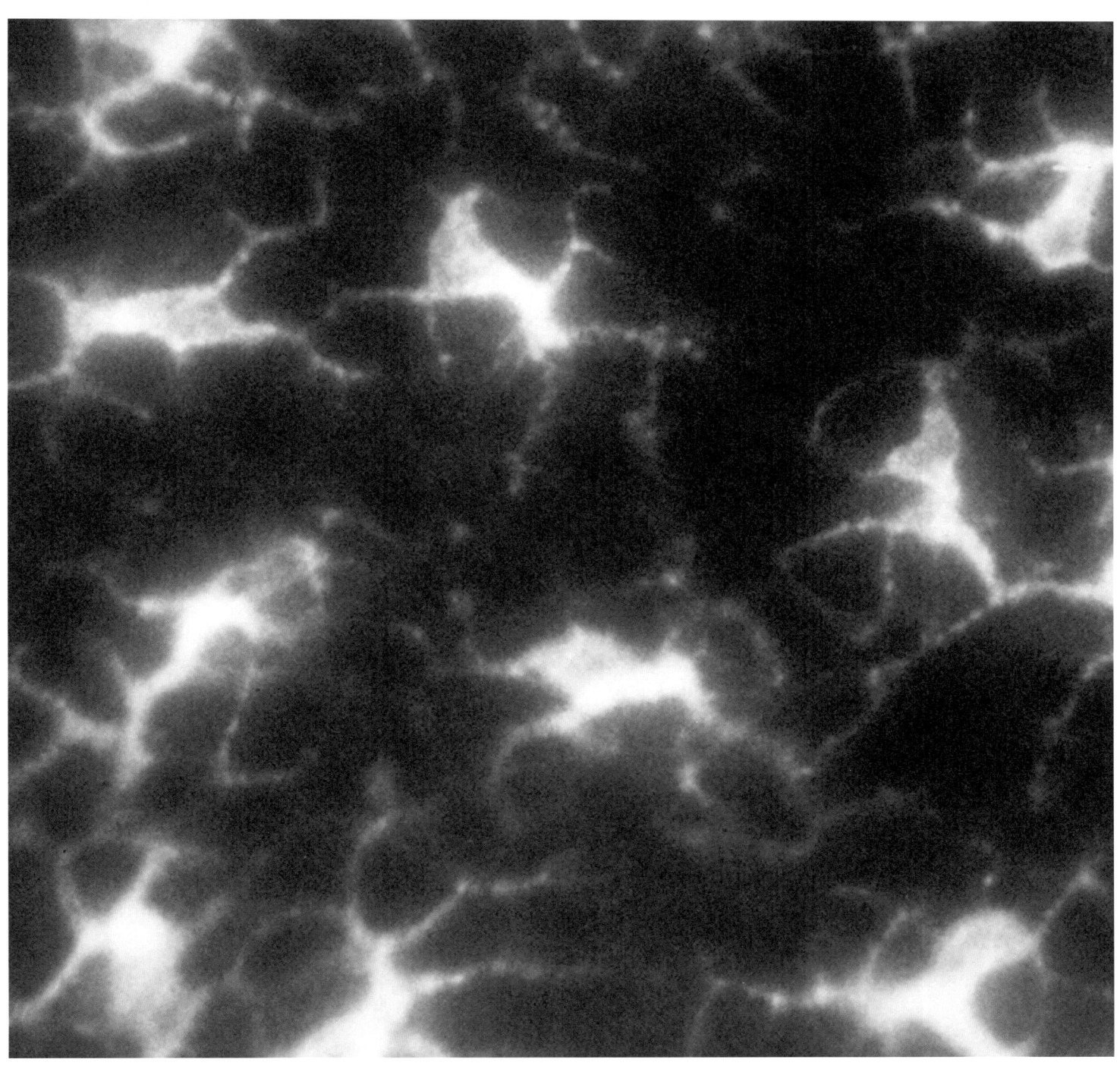

The Body Electric

Electrical signals play many roles in the body. They set the rhythm of the heart, generate other muscle contractions and nerve impulses, and regulate hormone secretion. The signals are generated by ions—electrically charged atoms—passing through pores in the membranes of cells.

These pores, or ion channels, are the research focus of molecular neurobiologist Roderick MacKinnon. Each channel consists of a single protein molecule, precisely folded to funnel the ions through. In 1998 MacKinnon's laboratory published the first three-dimensional image of the potassium ion channel, hailed as a "breakthrough of the year" in the journal *Science*.

The discovery also garnered MacKinnon an Albert Lasker Award for Basic Medical Research, the nation's most distinguished honor for outstanding contributions to basic and clinical medical research.

Viewing the architecture of the ion channel is important to understanding its function; it reveals how a balance of electrical forces and chemical bonds allows potassium ions through while blocking other ions. And basic knowledge revealed by MacKinnon's research may play an important role in the development of drugs to deal with diseases ranging from diabetes to heart problems.

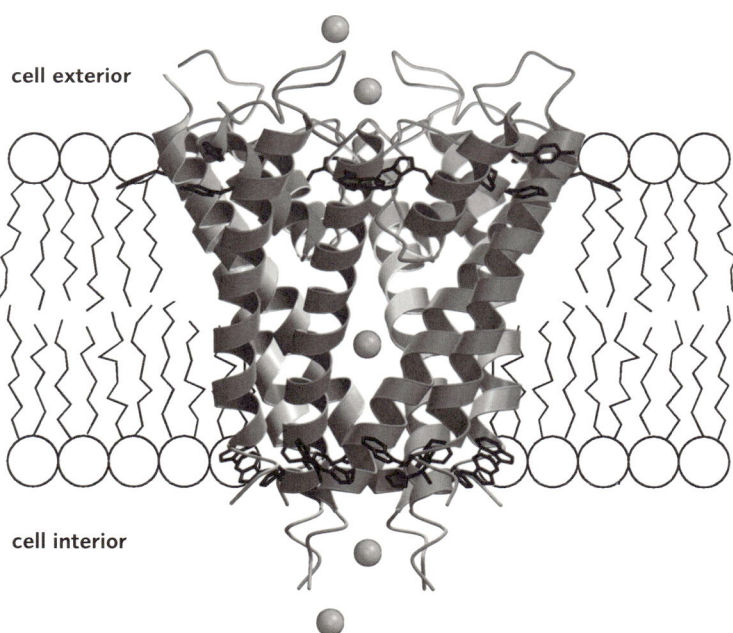

Diagram of a potassium channel embedded in a cell membrane. Potassium ions inside the cell flow out through the channel.

Roderick MacKinnon heads the laboratory of molecular neurobiology and biophysics.

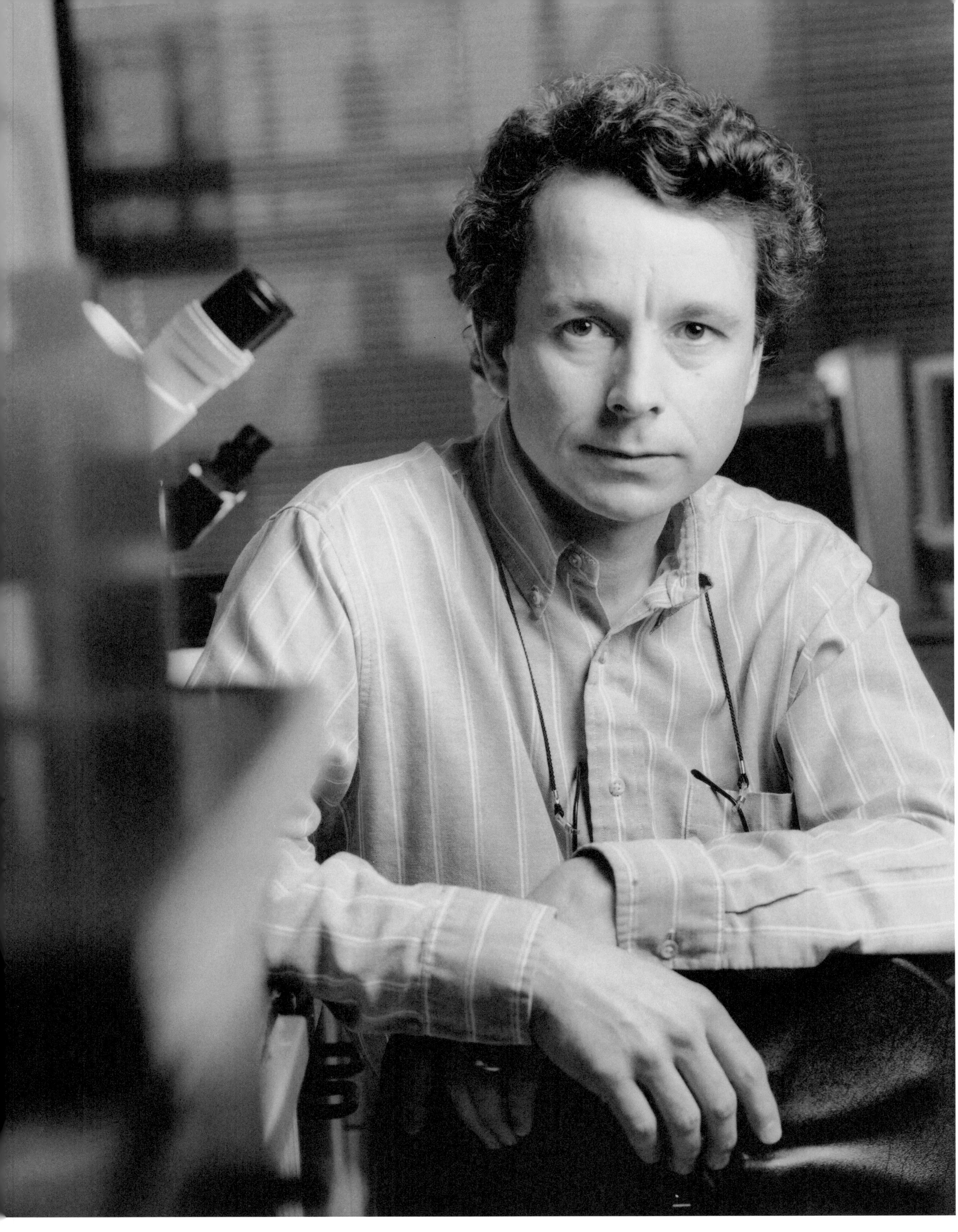

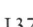

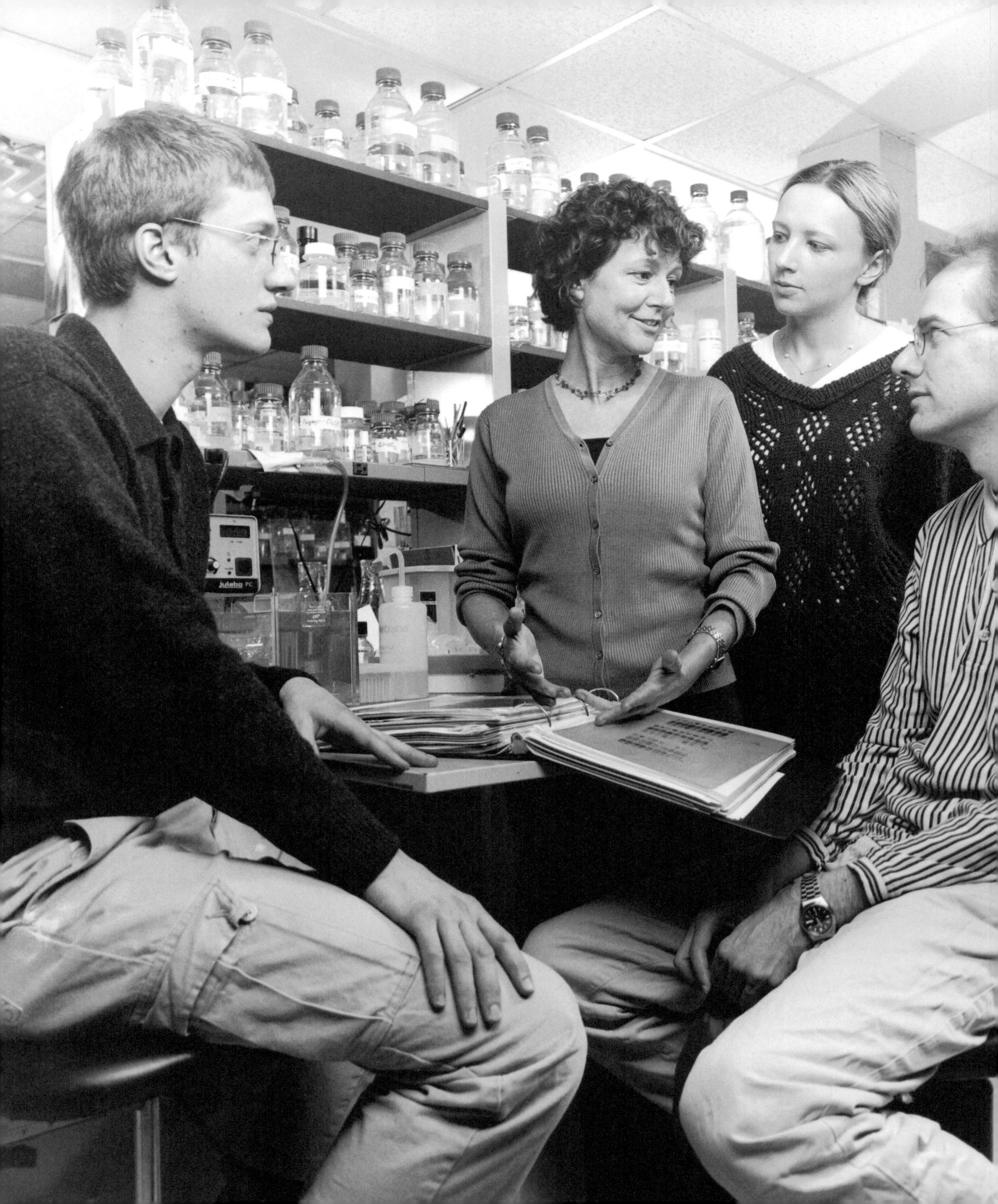

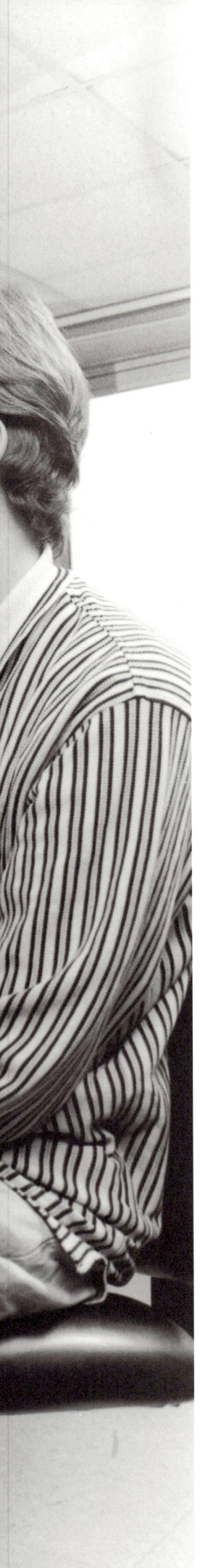

Chromosomal End Game

The chromosomes inside a cell's nucleus are long strands of DNA. The cell has mechanisms for repairing and maintaining the chromosomal DNA should it become damaged or broken. But scientists have long wondered how the cell knows that the end of a chromosome is its terminus and not a broken piece that needs mending. Cell biologist Titia de Lange studies these chromosome ends, which are called telomeres.

With her collaborator Jack Griffith at the University of North Carolina she has overturned conventional wisdom about the structure of telomeres. De Lange and Griffith discovered that chromosome ends are not blunt; rather, they are neatly looped, a finding that explains why the cell does not mistake telomeres for broken ends and provides insight into the cellular processes of cancer and aging.

Telomeres act something like the cap on a shoelace—they prevent the end of the DNA from becoming frayed—and the length of a cell's telomeres corresponds to its stage in life. In a cell from an infant, for example, the telomeres are long. With each cycle of cell division, however, a cell's telomeres are shortened a notch. And after about 50 divisions—when the telomeres have become too truncated to protect the DNA, perhaps because they can no longer form loops—the cell usually dies.

Recent experiments have shown that if scientists prevent the shortening of the telomeres, a cell can live and divide almost indefinitely. But this ability to make individual cells immortal does not necessarily point the way to a fountain of youth. Rather, scientists use it as a tool for understanding disease.

"In the case of cancer," observes de Lange, "a cell's suicide mechanism is actually something that protects us, that keeps a tumor from growing. So at the cellular level, there's a problem with immortality."

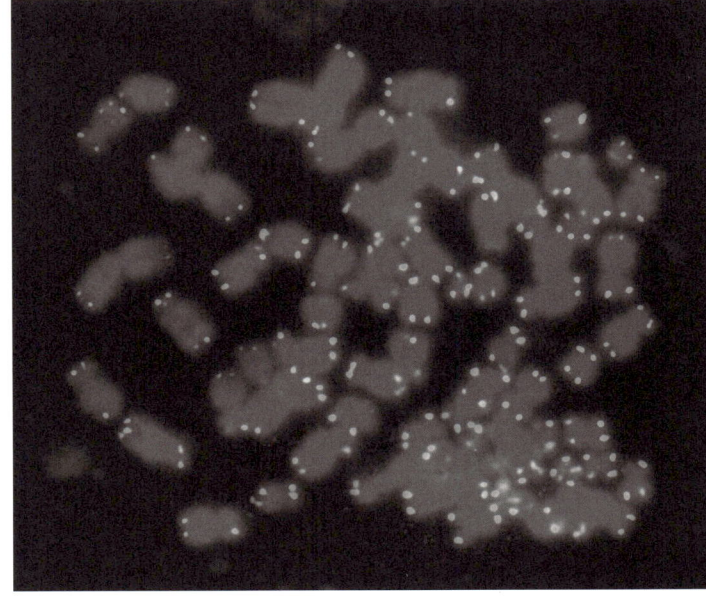

Telomeres appear as dots at the ends of chromosomes (right). In the laboratory of cell biology and genetics, from left: Dirk Hockemeyer, Titia de Lange, Agata Smogorzewska, Mark van Breugel.

The Chemistry of Life

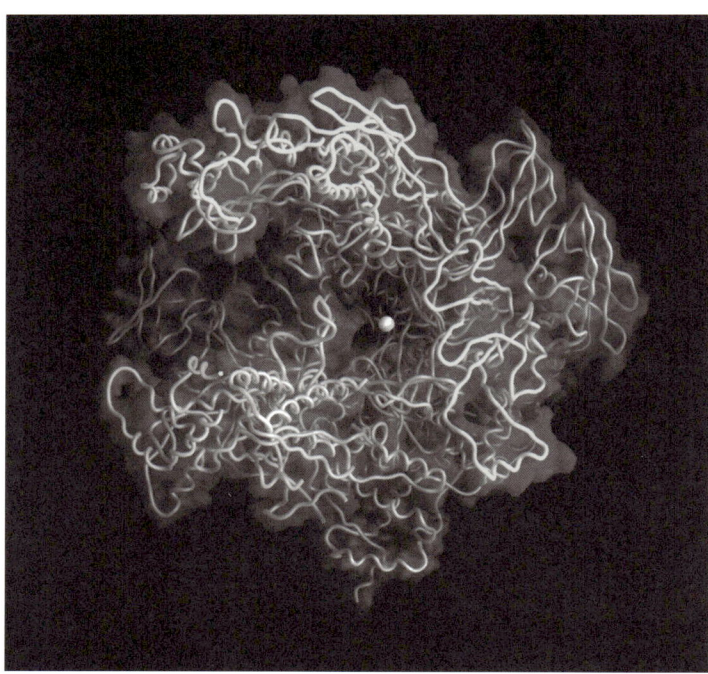

Seth Darst, head of a laboratory of molecular biophysics, solved the three-dimensional structure of cellular RNA polymerase, a molecular machine that activates individual genes by reading out the instructions encoded in their DNA.

If biology entered the age of the gene in the final years of the 20th century, at the beginning of the 21st century it is embarking on the age of the protein. Genes encode instructions for proteins, and gene sequences—the result, for example, of the human genome project—give scientists blueprint descriptions of proteins.

But proteins are not inert and flat like blueprints—they are complicated three-dimensional objects with protrusions, pockets, and electrical charges whose structure provides insight into their function. Because of this complexity it takes chemists, biologists, and others working together to discover what proteins do in a cell—how they form communication networks, for example, with regular routes for delivering chemical signals.

One way proteins communicate is by hooking up to each other in a sort of "molecular handshake," says biophysicist John Kuriyan. Kuriyan has solved the three-dimensional structure of an important protein involved in understanding cancer.

Synthetic chemists build on the knowledge of protein structures to tailor-make molecules that can enter such protein handshakes. The newly synthesized molecules thus block or alter normal protein activities and may be useful as drugs.

Rockefeller has long been home to distinguished chemists who study proteins. Today they collaborate more closely with biologists than ever before, bringing insights to bear on problems in genetics, neurobiology, cancer, and AIDS research.

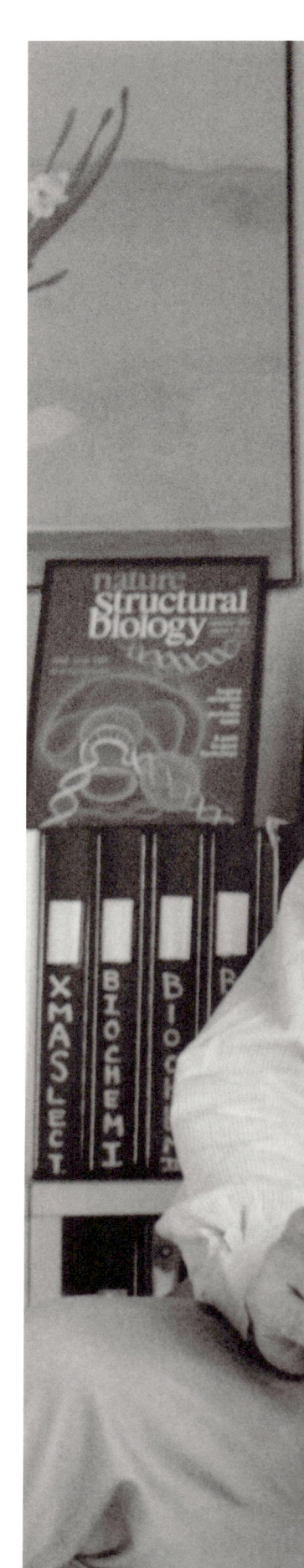

Robert Roeder (left) and Stephen Burley have collaborated to solve the three-dimensional structures of molecules important in converting DNA's instructions into proteins.

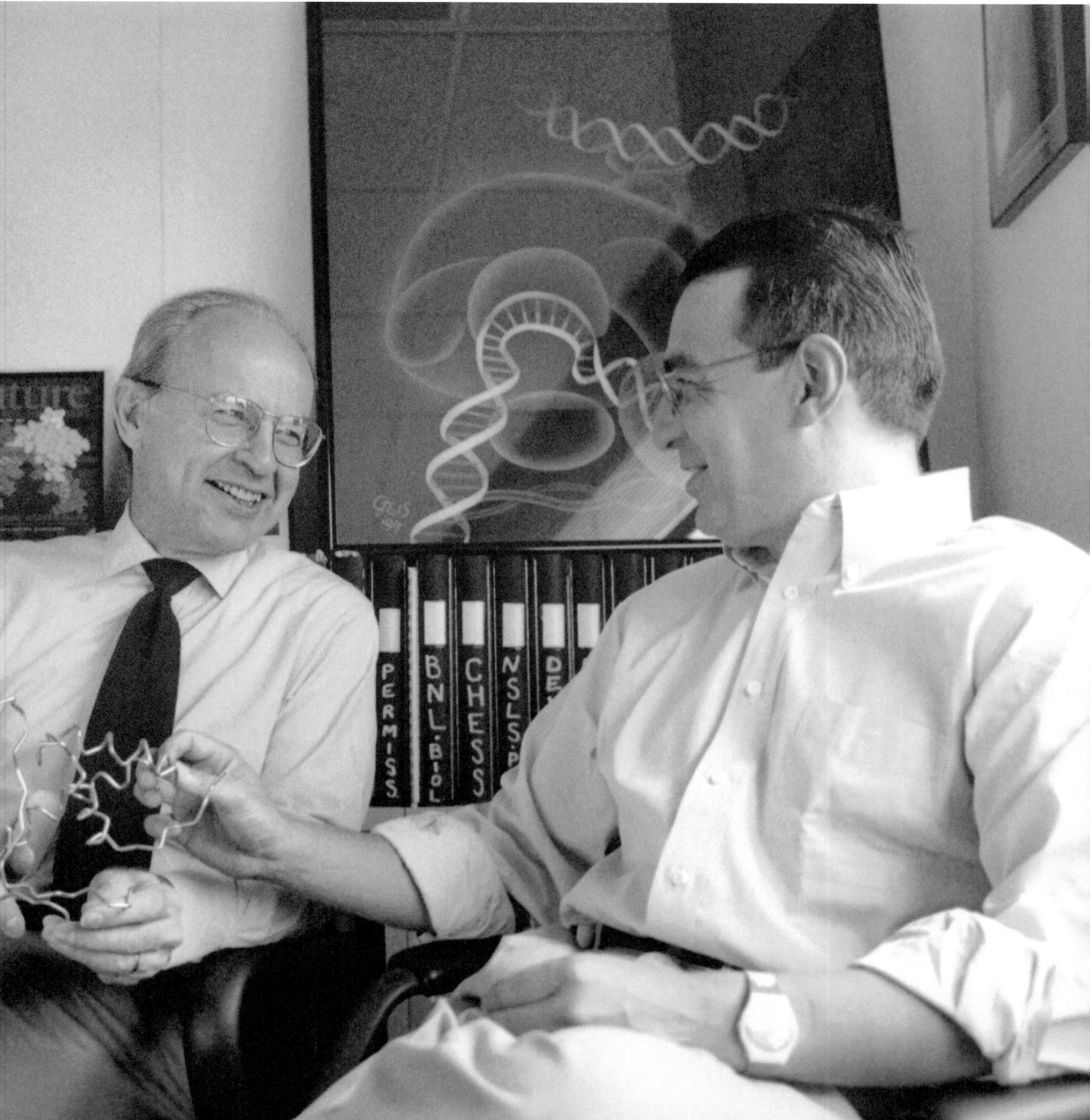

EPILOGUE

by David Rockefeller
Life Trustee and Honorary Chairman of the Board

During the early years of his long life, my grandfather had personal and painful experience with the devastating impact of infectious disease. His youngest sister died before the age of two, and his second child, Alice, succumbed when she was only one year old. Both deaths resulted from unknown and barely comprehended "childhood diseases." Losses such as these were commonplace for my grandfather's generation as they had been for all of recorded history. The "Angel of Death" hovered over every home across the world. I think we need look no further to understand why my grandfather responded to Frederick T. Gates' suggestion that work in the area of public health and medicine be added to his growing list of philanthropies.

The institution that resulted from Grandfather's experience and generosity, The Rockefeller Institute for Medical Research—today The Rockefeller University— has remained at the center of my family's philanthropy for more than a century. My father cared deeply about the Institute. He had a strong faith in science and believed that fundamental research into the mysteries of the human body would produce lasting and beneficial consequences for human society. He passed on his belief in that idea and his commitment to this institution to his children.

When I joined the Board of Trustees in 1940, it was an inspiration for me to work with Father in his capacity as president of the board. I observed the meticulous and caring way in which he followed the affairs of the Institute and the businesslike manner in which he presided at meetings.

When Father retired and I became president of the Board in 1949, it seemed to me that we needed to take a good hard look at the institution as it approached its 50th anniversary. I thought the review should include a thorough examination of its long list of accomplishments, where it stood in relation to other research institutions in this country and abroad, and where it ought to be going in the future. We decided at the outset to explore every possibility, including closing down the Institute. We asked Dr. Detlev Bronk, then the president of Johns Hopkins University and chairman of the policy-making committee of the National Science Foundation, in many ways the most distinguished American man of science of his day, to lead the review. It was a most fortunate choice.

The study took almost three years to complete, and it examined every conceivable aspect of the Institute—finances, endowment, governance, board leadership, scientific capacity, and the directions in which research in the medical and biological sciences were trending. As the process continued, two basic points became quite clear. First, the Rockefeller still had important scientific contributions to make, after the necessary organizational changes were implemented. And second, Detlev Bronk was the best man to lead the Institute into the future. As president of the Board, I asked him to leave Johns Hopkins University and come to Rockefeller. Much to my delight, Bronk accepted. During the next 15 years, it was Det's vision of a graduate university awarding the Ph.D. to a select group of promising young researchers that was implemented. This was, in some ways, a complete break with the past. In place of individual, and oftentimes isolated, laboratories headed by senior scientists, Det created a campus complete with students, dormitories, and even a faculty club. These were not just superficial amenities; they were essential in producing a collaborative intellectual atmosphere, where exciting and innovative science could flourish. Detlev Bronk's vision of 50 years ago has been gloriously achieved, and the nurturing of new scientific talent has continued.

At the same time that Bronk implemented these fundamental reforms, he also maintained the most important traditions. He hired outstanding faculty to ensure that the University would be a leader in all the fields of research represented. In this way, he continued the work of my grandfather and father, and those, especially William H. Welch and Simon Flexner, who had played the key roles in organizing the Institute. That founding group had designed an institution that would assemble the most qualified scientists and provide them with ideal conditions in which to work. Their emphasis, from the start, had been on people—outstanding people who could be expected to do great things. Bronk and his successors—Frederick Seitz, Joshua Lederberg, David Baltimore, Torsten Wiesel and, now, Arnold Levine, have maintained and even sharpened that first and strongest tradition at Rockefeller.

It is a history familiar to us all, but I think there are still lessons for us to learn. The Rockefeller University has always been an experimental model of excellence. It is "experimental" because like science itself, the institution should constantly change based on experience. By "excellence" I mean the pursuit of the best a human being or an institution is capable of in any realm of endeavor—the contribution to the sum of things. Excellence implies the highest standards of achievement against which individuals and societies can and should measure themselves.

At The Rockefeller University, the results have far outstripped the promise. Looking back on the experience of this single institution over the short span of 100 years, it is plain to see what benefits can result from supporting and encouraging research and education. Twenty Nobel Prizes awarded to Rockefeller scientists from Alexis Carrel in 1912 to Günter Blobel in 1999 testify to our extraordinary and ongoing accomplishments. Today's discoveries about heart disease, cancer, tuberculosis, and other diseases are leading to new treatments. In the next century, we will continue our essential work—nurturing excellence in science for the benefit of humankind.

ENDNOTES

Page 11   On pneumonia, see William Osler, *The Principles and Practice of Medicine*, seventh edition, New York: D. Appleton, 1909

Pages 11-12   Frederick Taylor Gates, *Chapters in My Life*, New York: The Free Press, 1977, pp. 181-182

Page 15   William H. Welch to Seth Low, President, Columbia University, November 5, 1900. Rockefeller Foundation Archives, R.B. Fosdick History of the Foundation, b. 40

Page 19   Simon Flexner to William H. Welch, April 8, 1902. Rockefeller Foundation Archives, Office of the Messrs. Rockefeller, b. 41

Page 20   Simon Flexner to Susan Dows Herter, August 3, 1913, quoted in George W. Corner, *A History of the Rockefeller Institute: 1901-1953, Origins and Growth*, New York: The Rockefeller Institute Press, 1964, p. 74

Page 22   Simon Flexner to William H. Welch, op. cit.

Page 26   Simon Flexner, "Sketch of the First Twenty-Five Years of The Rockefeller Institute for Medical Research," Rockefeller University Archives, RG 534U, b. 1

Page 45   Simon Flexner is quoted in Ron Chernow, *Titan: The Life of John D. Rockefeller, Sr.*, New York: Random House, 1998, pp. 474-475

Page 51   Simon Flexner, "Sketch of the First Twenty-Five Years," op. cit.

Page 52   Jacques Loeb is quoted in George W. Corner, *A History*, p. 80; Paul de Kruif, *The Sweeping Wind*, New York: Harcourt, Brace and World, 1962, p. 16; Alfred E. Cohn, *No Retreat From Reason and Other Essays*, New York: Harcourt, Brace, and Company, 1948, p. 263

Page 59   Oswald Avery's letter to his brother Roy, dated May 26, 1943, is transcribed in René J. Dubos, *The Professor, the Institute, and DNA*, New York: The Rockefeller University Press, 1976, pp. 217-220

Page 62   Albert Claude, "The Coming of Age of the Cell," *Science* 1975 (August 9), vol. 189, p. 433

Page 64   Paul de Kruif, *The Sweeping Wind*, op. cit.

Page 68   René Dubos is quoted in Carol L. Moberg, "Friend of the Good Earth," *Research Profiles No. 34* (summer 1989), The Rockefeller University Public Information Office

Page 72   Storm Van Leeuwen to Simon Flexner, quoted in Simon Flexner, "Karl Landsteiner, 1868-1943, Memorial Minute," typescript, files of The Rockefeller University, Office of Public Affairs; see also Peyton Rous, "Karl Landsteiner, 1868-1943," in *Obituary Notices of Fellows of the Royal Society, 1945-1948*, vol. 5, London: Morrison & Gibb, Ltd., pp. 295-324

Page 75   Herbert S. Gasser, "Medical Research: A Look Ahead at The Rockefeller Institute for Medical Research," Rockefeller Foundation Archives, Rockefeller Institute, Rockefeller Boards, 31.1, b. 44

Page 83   Herbert S. Gasser, "Medical Research," op. cit.

Page 86   Detlev Bronk, "The Conferring of Degrees: Opening Remarks," in *Occasional Papers of The Rockefeller Institute*, No. Eight, New York: The Rockefeller Institute Press, pp. 1-2

Page 89   Harrison's remarks are quoted in "New Buildings Are Dedicated and Cornerstones Are Unveiled," *Rockefeller Institute Quarterly* 1959, vol. 3, no. 2, p. 10

Page 108   Stanford Moore is quoted in "Elegant Molecules," *Research Profiles No. 8* (spring 1982), The Rockefeller University Public Information Office

Page 112   Detlev W. Bronk, "Science Advice in the White House," *Science* 1974 (October 11), vol. 186, pp. 116-121; Detlev W. Bronk, "The National Science Foundation: Origins, Hopes, and Aspirations," *Science* 1975 (May 2), vol. 188, pp. 409-414; Frank Brink Jr., "Detlev Wulf Bronk," *U.S. National Academy of Sciences Biographical Memoirs*, vol. 50, Washington, D.C., National Academy of Sciences, 1979, pp. 3-87

ACKNOWLEDGMENTS

The faculty, students, alumni, and staff of The Rockefeller University are passionate about science and justifiably proud of their institution. Their intimate knowledge of the University and their generosity in explaining the details of their work and sharing stories about the past have made this book possible. In addition, I am grateful for the unique insights into the institution's origins and growth offered by David Rockefeller and his staff. Members of The Rockefeller University Centennial Planning Committee guided the book's evolution from concept to publication. Joshua Lederberg kindly commented on a draft of the manuscript. Support from the Office of the President and the Public Affairs Office ensured its timely completion.

The University is fortunate to have its records preserved at the Rockefeller Archive Center. These include thousands of photographs, only a few of which have been reproduced here. Special thanks are due to all of the Archive Center staff, in particular the center's director Darwin Stapleton.

—Elizabeth Hanson

The Rockefeller Archive Center, located in Sleepy Hollow, New York, is a division of The Rockefeller University. In addition to the University's archives its collections include the archives of the Rockefeller family, the Rockefeller Foundation, the Rockefeller Brothers Fund, and other institutions, and the papers of associated individuals.

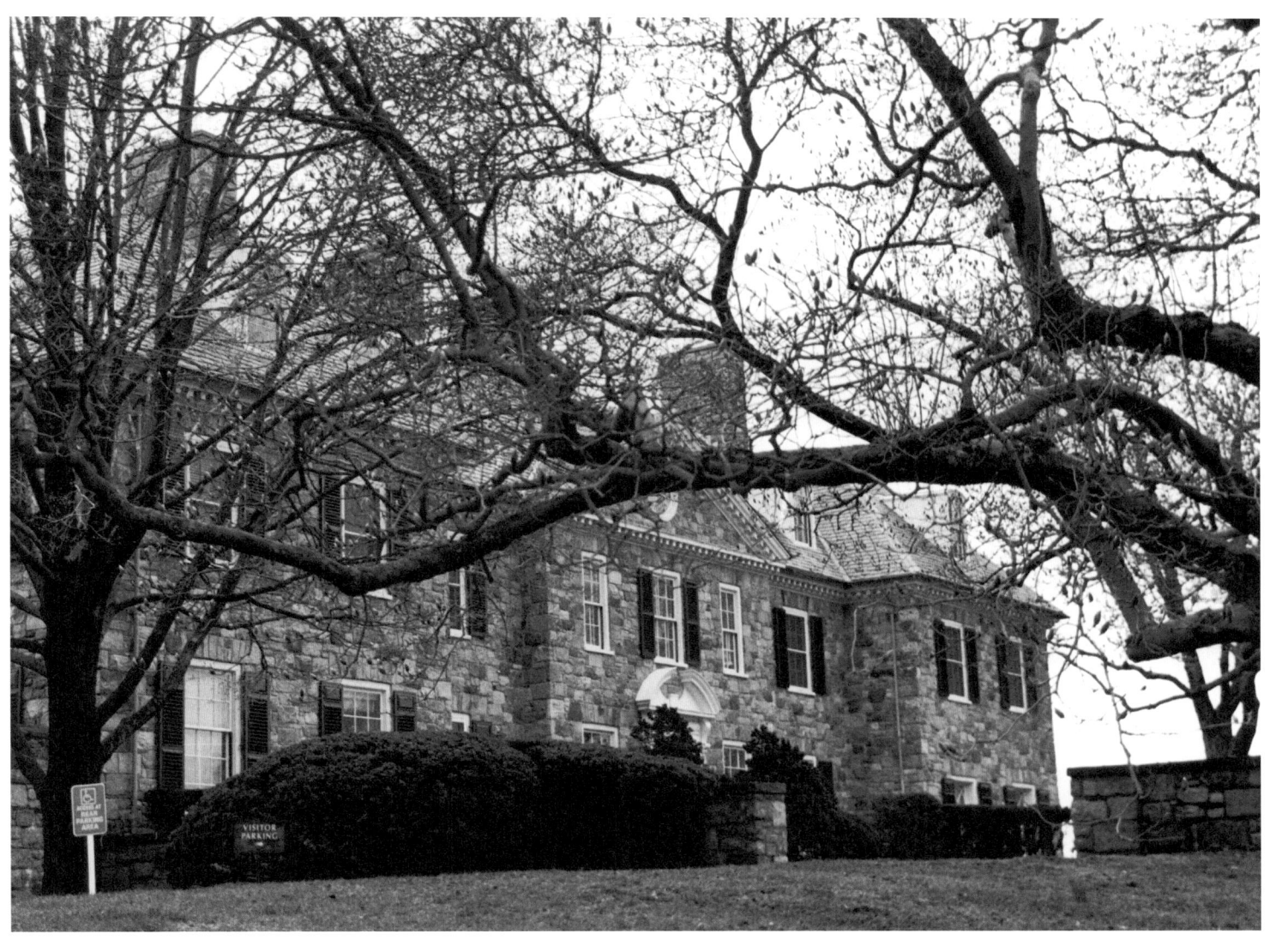

FACULTY OF THE ROCKEFELLER UNIVERSITY

The people listed below have been Members of the Institute, Professors of the University, or tenured Associate Professors of the University as of May 1, 2000. Asterisks (*) indicate members of the National Academy of Sciences; daggers (†) indicate Nobel laureates; double daggers (‡) indicate tenured Associate Professors.

Agosta, William C.
1963–1998; emeritus
1998–present

*Ahrens, Edward H., Jr.
1946–1985; emeritus
1985–present

Allfrey, Vincent G.
1941–1946; 1949–1991

Archibald, Reginald M.
1940–1980; emeritus
1980–present

Asanuma, Hiroshi
1972–1996; emeritus
1996–present

*Avery, Oswald T.
1913–1943; emeritus 1943–1955

*†Baltimore, David
President 1990–1992

*Bearn, Alexander G.
1951–1966

Bég, Mirza A.B.
1964–1990

Bergmann, Max
1934–1944

Berlin, Theodore H.
1961–1962

*†Blobel, Günter
1967–present

*Braun, Armin C.
1938–1981; emeritus
1981–1986

*Breslow, Jan L.
1984–present

*Brink, Frank Jr.
1953–1981; emeritus
1981–present

*Bronk, Detlev W.
President 1953–1968; emeritus
1968–1975

Brown, Wade Hampton
1913–1942

Burley, Steven K.
1990–present

†Carrel, Alexis
1906–1939; emeritus 1939–1944

Carter, D. Martin
1981–1993

*Case, Kenneth M.
1969–1988; emeritus
1988–present

*Cerami, Anthony
1969–1991

Chait, Brian T.
1979–present

*Chase, Merrill W.
1932–1976; emeritus
1976–present

*Choppin, Purnell W.
1957–1985

Chua, Nam-Hai
1971–present

Cohen, E.G.D.
1963–1993; emeritus
1993–present

*Cohen, Joel E.
1975–present

Cohn, Alfred E.
1911–1944; emeritus 1944–1957

*Cohn, Zanvil A.
1958–1993

Cole, Michael
1969–1978

*Cole, Rufus
1909–1937; emeritus 1937–1944

‡Connelly, Clarence
1954–1984; emeritus
1984–present

*Cool, Rodney L.
1970–1988

*Craig, Lyman C.
1933–1974

Cranefield, Paul F.
1966–1996; emeritus
1996–present

Cross, Frederick R.
1989–present

Cross, George A.M.
1982–present

Cunningham, Bruce A.
1966–1992

*Darnell, James E., Jr.
1974–present

Darst, Seth
1992–present

Davidson, Donald H.
1970–1976

*†de Duve, Christian R.
1962–1988; emeritus
1988–present

de Lange, Titia
1990–present

DiNardo, Stephen
1988–1998

*Dobzhansky, Theodosius
1962–1975

*Dole, Vincent P.
1941–1983; emeritus
1983–present

*Dubos, René J.
1927–1942; 1944–1982

*†Edelman, Gerald M.
1960–1992

Edelstein, Ludwig
1960–1965

*Estes, William K.
1968–1979

*Farquhar, Marilyn G.
1970–1973

*Feigenbaum, Mitchell J.
1987–present

Feinberg, Joel
1967–1977

Field, Frank H.
1970–1989; emeritus
1989–present

Fischetti, Vincent A.
1970–present

Fishman, Jack
1980–1988

*Flexner, Simon
Director 1903–1935; emeritus
1935–1946

Frankfurt, Harry G.
1963–1976

Friedman, Jeffrey M.
1980–present

Gadsby, David C.
1975–present

*†Gasser, Herbert S.
Director 1935–1953; emeritus
1953–1963

Gilbert, Charles D.
1983–present

*Glimm, James
1974–1982

*Goebel, Walther F.
1924–1970; emeritus 1970–1993

*Gotschlich, Emil C.
1960–present

148

Goulianos, Konstantin A.
1971–present

*Granick, Sam
1939–1977

*Greengard, Paul
1983–present

‡Gregory, John D.
1957–1991

*Griffin, Donald R.
1965–1986; *emeritus*
1986–present

*Hanafusa, Hidesaburo
1973–1999; *emeritus*
1999–present

*†Hartline, H. Keffer
1953–1974; *emeritus* 1974–1983

Hatten, Mary Elizabeth
1992–present

Heintz, Nathaniel
1983–present

Hemmati-Brivanlou, Ali
1994–present

*Hirsch, James G.
1950–1981

Hirsch, Jules
1954–1998; *emeritus*
1998–present

Ho, David
1996–present

Hoagland, Charles L.
1937–1946

*Horsfall, Frank L., Jr.
1934–1937; 1941–1960

*Hotchkiss, Rollin D.
1935–1982; *emeritus*
1982–present

*Hudspeth, A. James
1995–present

*Jacobs, Walter A.
1907–1949; *emeritus* 1949–1967

‡Jesaitus, Margeris
1950–1986

*Kac, Mark
1961–1984

*Kaiser, Emil Thomas
1982–1988

Kappas, Attallah
1966–present

Khuri, Nicola N.
1968–present

‡King, Te Piao
1953–2000; *emeritus*
2000–present

Knight, Bruce Jr.
1961–present

*Krause, Richard M.
1954–1975

Kreek, Mary Jeanne
1964–present

Kripke, Saul A.
1973–1977

*Kunitz, Moses
1913–1953; *emeritus* 1953–1978

*Kunkel, Henry G.
1945–1983

*Kunkel, Louis O.
1931–1949; *emeritus* 1949–1960

Kuriyan, John
1987–present

*Lancefield, Rebecca C.
1918–1965; *emeritus* 1965–1981

*†Landsteiner, Karl
1922–1939; *emeritus* 1939–1943

*†Lederberg, Joshua
President 1978–1990; *emeritus*
1990–present

*Levene, P.A.T.
1905–1939; *emeritus* 1930–1940

*Levine, Arnold J.
President 1998–present

Libchaber, Albert J.
1994–present

*†Lipmann, Fritz A.
1957–1969; *emeritus* 1969–1986

*Lloyd, David P.C.
1939–1943, 1946–1970; *emeritus*
1970–1985

Loeb, Jacques
1910–1924

*Longsworth, Lewis G.
1928–1970; *emeritus* 1970–1981

*Lorente de Nó, Rafael
1936–1970; *emeritus* 1970–1990

Luck, David J.L.
1962–1998

*MacInnes, Duncan A.
1926–1950; *emeritus* 1950–1965

*MacKinnon, Roderick
1996–present

‡Manning, James
1967–1996; *emeritus*
1996–present

*Marler, Peter R.
1966–1989; *emeritus*
1989–present

Martin, Donald A.
1967–1977

Mauro, Alexander
1959–1989

Mauzerall, David C.
1954–present

*McCarty, Maclyn
1940–1981; *emeritus*
1981–present

*McEwen, Bruce S.
1966–present

*McKean, Henry P., Jr.
1966–1970

*McMaster, Philip D.
1919–1963; *emeritus* 1963–1973

*Meltzer, Samuel J.
1904–1920

*†Merrifield, R. Bruce
1949–1992; *emeritus*
1992–present

*Michaelis, Leonor
1929–1940; *emeritus* 1940–1949

*Miller, George A.
1967–1981

*Miller, Neal E.
1966–1980; *emeritus*
1980–present

*Mirsky, Alfred E.
1927–1971; *emeritus* 1971–1974

Model, Peter
1967–2000; *emeritus*
2000–present

*†Moore, Stanford
1939–1982

Müller, Miklos
1964–present

*Murphy, James B.
1910–1950

‡Murphy, James S.
1951–1989; *emeritus*
1989–present

Noguchi, Hideyo
1904–1928

*†Northrop, John H.
1915–1962; *emeritus* 1962–1987

*Nottebohm, Fernando
1967–present

Nuzzenzweig, Michel C.
1989–present

O'Donnell, Michael
1996–present

Olitsky, Peter K.
1917–1952; *emeritus* 1952–1964

*Opie, Eugene L.
1904–1910 (*Affiliate* 1941–1971)

*Osterhout, W.J.V.
1925–1939; *emeritus* 1939–1964

Ott, Jürg
1996–present

*Pais, Abraham
1963–1988; *emeritus*
1988–present

*†Palade, George E.
1946–1973

Perlmann, Gertrude E.
1946–1974

*Pfaff, Donald W.
1966–present

*Pfaffman, Carl
1965–1983; *emeritus* 1983–1994

*Porter, Keith R.
1939–1961

*Ratliff, Floyd
1954–1989; *emeritus* 1989–1999

Ravetch, Jeffrey V.
1996–present

‡Reeke, George
1970–present

Reich, Edward
1962–1984

Rice, Charles M.
2000–present

*Rivers, Thomas M.
1922–1955; *emeritus*
1955–1962

‡Rizack, Martin A.
*1960–1990; emeritus
1990–present*

*Roeder, Robert G.
1982–present

*Rota, Gian-Carlo
1965–1967

Rothen, Alexandre
1927–1970; emeritus 1970–1987

*†Rous, Peyton
1909–1945; emeritus 1945–1970

*Sabin, Florence R.
1925–1938; emeritus 1938–1953

Sakmar, Thomas P.
1990–present

‡Sassa, Shigeru
*1968–2000; emeritus
2000–present*

‡Schoenfeld, Robert L.
*1957–1990; emeritus
1990–present*

‡Schreiber, Morris
1962–1988

*Seitz, Frederick
*President 1968–1978; emeritus
1978–present*

*Shannon, James A.
1970–1975

*Shedlovsky, Theodore
1927–1969; emeritus 1969–1976

*Shope, Richard E.
1925–1949, 1952–1966

*Siekevitz, Philip
*1954–1988; emeritus
1988–present*

Siggia, Eric
1997–present

*Smith, Theobald
1919–1929; emeritus 1929–1934

‡Spector, Leonard B.
*1960–1989; emeritus
1989–present*

*†Stanley, Wendell M.
1931–1948

*†Stein, William H.
1937–1980

Steinman, Ralph M.
1970–present

Stoffel, Markus
1995–present

Stoll, Norman R.
1927–1963; emeritus 1963–1976

Swift, Homer F.
*1910–1914, 1919–1946;
emeritus 1946–1953*

*Tamm, Igor
1949–1992; emeritus 1992–1995

*†Tatum, Edward L.
1957–1975

TenBroeck, Carl
*1915–1920, 1927–1951; emeritus
1951–1966*

Tomasz, Alexander
1961–present

*Trager, William
*1933–1980; emeritus
1980–present*

*Uhlenbeck, George E.
1961–1974; emeritus 1974–1988

*Van Slyke, Donald D.
1907–1948; emeritus 1948–1971

Wang, Hao
1966–1991

Webster, Leslie T.
1920–1943

*Weiss, Paul A.
1954–1964; emeritus 1964–1989

*†Wiesel, Torsten N.
*1983–1992; President
1992–1998; emeritus
1998–present*

Wilson, Victor J.
1956–present

‡Wood, Henry N.
*1955–1990; emeritus
1990–present*

*Woolley, D. Wayne
1939–1966

Young, Michael W.
1978–present

‡Zabriskie, John B.
*1960–2000; emeritus
2000–present*

*Zinder, Norton D.
*1952–1999; emeritus
1999–present*

INDEX

Page numbers in *italics* refer to illustrations.

A

Aaron Diamond AIDS Research Center, 124
Abby Aldrich Rockefeller Hall, *88, 89, 90*, 91
Academic Council, 95
addiction research, 105
Adrian, E.D., 112
African sleeping sickness, 34, 35
Ahrens, Edward H., Jr., 106
AIDS, 102, 124, 134
Albert Lasker Award for Basic Medical Research, 116, 136
Albert, Matthew, 130, *130*
Albertini, Marcus, *124*
Alfinsen, Christian B., 108
alumni, 92, *94-95*, 96, *97*, *100-101*, 103, 106
Alzheimer's disease, 122
ambulance, *36*
amino acids, protein structure and, 108, 111
Animal and Plant Pathology, Department of, *24*, 25-26, 70, 84
animals, diseases of, 25-26, 76, 84
antibiotics, 57, 59, 68, 122-123
antibodies, 72, 92
antigens, 72
antivivisection movement, 49
apolipoprotein E, 106
apparatus, scientific, 54, *78*, 79, *79*, *80*, *81*, *110*, 111
Arndt, William F., Jr., 100, *100-101*
Arrowsmith (Lewis), 31
atherosclerosis, 106
Avery, Oswald T., 7, 45, 54, *55*, 56-59, 68

B

Babers, Frank H., 57
bacteria
  antibiotic-resistant, 122-123
  in milk, 32
  pneumococcal, *45*, 56, 59
  streptococcal, 76
Baltimore, David, 96, *97*, 143
Barker, Bertha, *46-47*
Barr, Alfred, 89
Bennett, H. Stanley, 66
Bergmann, Max, 65, *65*, 108
Berlin, Ted, 92
Beth Israel Hospital, methadone maintenance clinic, *104*, 105

Bhardwaj, Nina, 134
Bhatt, Rhupal, *130*
Biggs, Hermann M., *10, 14*
bioinformatics, 117
biology, current research, 115-125
Blobel, Günter, 62, 118, *119*, 121-122
blood
  antigens, 72
  chemical analysis, 54
  fat transport, 106
  Lindbergh pump, 79
  plasma volume measurement, *80*
  preservation, 28
  typing, 72
boiler house, 42
Bonneville, Mary A., *100*
Breslow, Jan L., 106, 128
Bronk, Detlev W., *82-83*, 89, *100-101*, *112-113*
  academic philosophy, 86, 92
  addiction research support, 105
  future of Institute study, 85, 143
  grant procurement, 112
  legacy, 86, 89, 95
  presidency, 85-86, 89, 92, 100-101, 116
  science policy leadership role, 112-113
  student interviews, 85, 100-101
Burley, Stephen K., 123, *140-141*
Bush, Vannevar, 84

C

cancer, 7, 102, 133, 134, 138
Capellino, Frank, 36
Carnegie, Andrew, 39
Carnegie Institute, 39
Carrel, Alexis, 20, 28, *28-29*, 41, *41*, 68, 79
Caspary Hall and Auditorium, *82-83*, *87*, 91
Cebra, John J., *100*
cell biology, 7, 60, 62-63, *63*, 75, 79, 86, *114-115*, 121-122, 138
Center for Field Research in Ethology and Ecology, 92, 96
Center for the Study of Hepatitis C, 125
cerebrospinal meningitis, Flexner's serum, 34, 56
Chagas' disease, 124
chaos theory, 121
chemistry, interdisciplinary research, 116-117, 118, 121-123, 140
Chicago, University of, 12, 38, 39, 42
Chickering, Henry, 36

China Medical Board, 41
cholesterol research, 106
Choppin, Purnell, 36
chromatography, 106, 108
Claude, Albert, 60, *61*, 62, *94-95*
clinical research
  emphasis on, 25-26
  as envisioned by Cole, 25, 52, 54
  Gates on American practice, 11-13
  and the physical sciences, 52
Cohen, Joel, 124
Cohn, Alfred E., 45, 52
Cohn, Zanvil A., 134
Cole, Rufus, 25, 45, 52, 54, 56
computers, use of, 79, 96, 117
Convocations, 86, 130, *130-131*
Coolidge, Charles, 42
Cornell University Medical College, 95-96
countercurrent distribution apparatus, *81*
Craig, Lyman, 81

D

Dakin, Henry, 28
Darnell, James E., Jr., 133, *133*
Darnell, Robert B., 134
Darst, Seth, 140
de Duve, Christian, 60, 62, *94-95*
de Kruif, Paul, *30*, 31, 64
de Lange, Titia, *138-139*, 139
dendritic cells, 134, *134*, 135
development campaign, first, 95
diabetes research, 54, 128
diarrhea epidemics, 32
Directors, Board of. *See also* Scientific Directors, Board of; Trustees, Board of.
  appointment of first director, 19
  first, *10, 14, 15*, 19
  split, 22
Disease. *See* infectious disease; names of specific diseases.
DNA
  chip technology, 121, *132-133*
  discovery of function, 54-59
  research, 117, 118, 121, 133
  telomere role, 138
Dodge, Frederick A., Jr., *100*
Doetsch, Fiona, *130*
Dohrn, Anton, 22
Dole, Vincent, 105, 106
Doetsch, Fiona—
Dubos, René J., 57, *57*, 68, 95, 108
Dunn, M.S., 41
dysentery, 19, 28

E

Edelman, Gerald, 92, *94-95*
Edelstein, Ludwig, 92
Edmundson, Allen B., *100*
Eisenhower, Dwight D., *112*, 112-113
electrical signals, in human body, 136
electron micrograph, 62, *63*, 86
electron microscopy, 60, 62, 79
enzymes. *See* names of specific enzymes.
Erlanger, Joseph, 75
Europe, medical research in, 12, 22, 41, 65
Evolution and Organization of the University Clinic (Flexner), 49

F

faculty, 7, 95, 96, 116, 148-150. *See also* names of specific faculty members and of specific awards and prizes.
Faculty and Students Club, 91, 130
fat cells, 106
Feigenbaum, Mitchell J., 120
fibroblast, *63*
Fischer, Emil, 51
Flexner, Abraham, 49
Flexner, Simon, *10*, *18*, 28, 31, 36, 45, *48*
  cerebrospinal meningitis serum, 34
  laboratory, 20, *30*, 34
  legacy, 19, 26, 49, 64
  medical research views, 22, 51, 52, 116
  staff selection, 20, 41, 46, 49, 51, 52, 65, 72
  vision for Institute, 19-22, 124, 143
Flexner Hall, *42-43*
Founder's Hall, *16*, *17*, 42, *42-43*, *130-131*
Francis, Thomas, Jr., 57
free fatty acids, 106
Friedman, Jeffrey, 106, 128
Fullam, Ernest, 60

G

Gaasterland, Terry, *117*
gas gangrene, 28
Gasser, Herbert, 64, *74-75*, 75, 83, 84, 85
Gates, Frederick T., 7, 11-13, *18*, 22, 116
gene activators, 133
gene expression, 133

General Motors Cancer Research
  Foundation, 133
genetics, 96, 106, *114-115*, 117, 118,
  128, 140
genomes, 79
gentamicin, 123
Germany, medical research, 12,
  22, 65
Gilman, Daniel Coit, 86
glassblowing, 78, *78*
Goebel, Walter F., 45, *57*
Golden, William, 112
Goodner, Kenneth, *57*
Granit, Ragnar, *100*
Gratia, Leon E., 30
Greene, Lewis J., *100*
Greengard, Paul, 122
Griffin, Donald, 92
Griffith, Frederick, 59
Griffith, Jack, 138
Guam, 76, *76-77*
Gustav, King (of Sweden), *70-71*

H
hair cells, *123*
Hanafusa, Hidesaburo, 102
haptens, 72
Harrison and Abramovitz
  (architects), 89
Harrison, Wallace, 89
Hartline, H. Keffer, *85, 94-95*, 100
hearing, hair cell role, 123
heart, Lindbergh pump, 79
heart disease research, 106, 128
Heidelberger, Michael, 45, 56
hepatitis C, 122, 125
heroin addiction research, 105
Herter, Christian A., *14*, 15, 22, 25
Hirsch, Jules, 106
HIV, 122, 124, 134
Ho, David, 124
Hockemeyer, Dirk, *138-139*
Hodes, Horace L., *76-77*
hog cholera, 25
Holt, L. Emmett, *10, 14*, 15, 53
Holt, Steve, *76-77*
homeopathy, 13
hookworm eradication, 39
Hopkins, John W., III, *100*
Hotchkiss, Rollin, *57*
Howard Hughes Medical Institute,
  36, 96, 118
Hudspeth, A. James, 123
Hughes, Howard, 36
Hughes, Rupert, 36

I
immunochemistry, 72
immunology, 64, 72, 92, 134
infectious disease. *See also* names of
  specific diseases.
  early focus on, 25, 64
  germ theory, 12
  as leading cause of death, 11
  microbial detective work, 34-35
  resurgence, 122, 124
  war research, 28, 76
influenza, 54

instruments, scientific. *See*
  apparatus, scientific; names of
  specific instruments.
Intel Science Talent Search, 124
Interchemical Corporation, 60
International Geophysical Year,
  112, 113
International Health Board, 39
ion channel, 136, *136*

J
Jacobs, Walter, *21*
*Journal of Biophysical and
  Biochemical Cytology,* 66, *66*
Journal of Cell Biology, 66
Journal of Experimental Medicine,
  49, 66, 102
Journal of General Physiology, 66

K
Kac, Mark, 92, *93*
Kaiser Wilhelm Institute, 26, 65
Karayiorgou, Maria, 128
Kennedy, John F., *112-113*
Kiley, Dan, 91
Killian, James R., *112,* 113
Knight, Bruce, 85
Koch, Robert, 12
Koch Institute, 22
Kosrae, Micronesia, genetic
  research, 128
Kreek, Mary Jeanne, 105
Kunitz, Moses, 108
Kunkel, Henry, 92, *92*
Kuriyan, John, 102, 140

L
laboratories, *44-45, 46-47, 108*
  construction, 36
  Flexner, 20, 30, 34
  in Gasser administration, 75
  intellectual freedom allowed,
    8, 19-20, 22, 75
  interdisciplinary approach, 56, 86,
    92, 117, 130, 143
  Levene, 20-21, 53, 54
  Noguchi, 34-35
  number of, 64
  Rockefeller's visit to, 45
  role of, 8, 19-20, 64, 92
  untenured faculty, 96
Lacks, Sanford A., *100*
Lancefield, Rebecca, *76, 76*
Landsteiner, Karl, 72, *72-73*
Lederberg, Joshua, 96, *97,* 143
leptin, 106, 128
Levene, Phoebus A.T., 20, *20*, 41,
  53, 54
Levine, Arnold J., 7-9, *97, 98*, 117,
  121, 143
Lewis, Sinclair, 31, *31*
Libchaber, Albert, *120,* 121
Lindbergh, Charles, 79
lipids, 106
Lipmann, Fritz, 92, *94-95*
Loeb, Jacques, 20, 31, 41, *50-51,*
  51-52, 66
lysosome, 62

M
MacArthur Foundation, genius
  awards, 116
McCarty, Maclyn, *58,* 59
McCormick, John Rockefeller, 15
McFarlane, Karen, *124*
McKinney, John, 122
MacKinnon, Roderick, 136, *137*
McLean, Franklin C., 41
MacLeod, Colin M., 59
Manhattan House of Detention
  for Men, 105
Marler, Peter, 92
mathematics, 92, 121, 124
M.D.-Ph.D. program, 95-96
medical education, 49, 52
  in nineteenth century, 11-13
medical research
  current, 116-141
  Flexner's legacy, 19, 26, 49, 64
  Flexner's views on, 22, 51, 52, 116
  Gates' views on, 7, 11-13, 116
  growth of, 83
  interdisciplinary approach, 56, 86,
    92, 117, 121-124, 125, 130, 143
  in nineteenth century, 11-13
  and the physical sciences, 51-81,
    116
Meltzer, Samuel, 20, 41
meningitis, 28, 34
Merrifield, R. Bruce, 41, 111, *111*
metabolism studies, 105, 106
methadone, 105
methadone maintenance clinic, *104,*
  105
Meyer, Gustave, *21*
miasma, as cause of illness, 12
Microbe Hunters, The (de Kruif), 31
microbiology, 34-35
microsome, 60
microtome, 79
milk
  bacterial content, 32
  sampling, *32-33*
Millbrook, New York, Center for
  Field Research in Ethology and
  Ecology, 92, 96
Miller, Dorothy, 89
Mirsky, Alfred E., 95
molecular biology, 39, 54, 59, 96,
  102, 106, 118, 122-123, 133, 136
Moore, Stanford, 75, *94-95,* 108,
  108, 109
mortality
  meningitis, 34
  pneumococcal pneumonia, 56
  tuberculosis, 11, 122
Muir, Tom, 123
Murphy, James B., 60

N
Naples Zoological Station, 22
National Academy of Sciences,
  52, 112
National Medals of Science, 116
National Research Council, 41,
  49, 112
National Science Foundation,
  112, 143

Naval Research Unit, 76, *76-77*
Navas, Maria Angeles, *129*
neurobiological research, 85, 122,
  123, 136
New York City Board of Health
  cerebrospinal meningitis
    epidemic, 34
  milk study, 32, *33-34*
Nobel Prize
  award ceremony, *70-71,* 119
  Baltimore, David, 96, *97,* 143
  Blobel, 62, 118, *119,* 121-122
  Carrel, 20, 28, *28-29,* 41, *41,* 68, 79
  Claude, Albert, 60, *61,* 62, *94-95*
  de Duve, Christian, 60, 62, *94-95*
  Edelman, 92, *94-95*
  Gasser, 64, *74-75,* 75, 83, 84, 85
  Hartline, 85, *94-95,* 100
  Landsteiner, 72, *72-73*
  laureates, 51, 65, *94-95,* 95,
    116, 144
  Lederberg, 96, *97,* 143
  Lipmann, 92, *94-95*
  Merrifield, 41, 111, *111*
  Moore, 75, *94-95,* 108, *108, 109*
  Northrop, 26, 31, 70, *70-71*
  Palade, 60, 62, *62,* 86, *94-95,* 118
  Rous, 7, 28, 49, 102, *103*
  Stanley, 26, 70, *70-71*
  Stein, 75, 108, *108, 109*
  Tatum, 92
  Wiesel, 85, 96, *97,* 98, 143
Noguchi, Hideyo, 20, 34, 35, *35*
nonlinear dynamics, 121
Northrop, John H., 26, 31, 70, *70-71*
Novy, F. G., 31
Nurses Residence, *42-43*
Nyswander, Marie, 105, *105*

O
obese gene, 128
obesity research, 106, 128
O'Connor, Basil, *76-77*
Office of Scientific Research and
  Development, 112
Olitsky, Peter, 41
Opie, Eugene, 20, 46
Oppenheimer, Robert, 84
Oroya fever, 34
Osler, William, 11-12, 56
Osterhout, Suydam, *100-101*
Osterhout, W.J.V., 66
Oxford University, 49

P
p53 tumor suppressor gene,
  132-133, 133
Paasche, Eystein K.M., *100*
Pais, Abraham, 92
Palade, George, 60, 62, *62,* 86,
  94, 118
papilloma, 102
Papperitz, Wolfgang, *78*
Pasteur, Louis, 12
Pasteur Institute, 22, 51
Peachey, Lee D., *100-101, 100-101*
Pearce, Louise, 34, 35
Peking Union Medical College,
  40-41, 41

peptide synthesis, *110, 111*
Pfaffmann, Carl, 92
philanthropy
  patronage of science through, 39
  philosophy of John D. Rockefeller, 8, 38-39
  of Rockefeller family, 7, 15, 16, 22, 25, 26, 34, 125, 142
Philosopher's Garden, *91*
photometer, *80*
physics, 92, 117
plaque, protein, 122, *122*
pneumococcal bacteria, *45,* 56, 59
pneumonia, 11, 55, 56, 57, 59, 68
Porter, Keith, 60, 62, *62,* 66
potassium ion channel, 136, *136*
power house (building), 42
Princeton laboratories, *24-25, 25-26,* 70, 84
Principles and Practice of Medicine (Osler), 11-12
protein
  gene activators, 133
  plaque accumulation, 122, *122*
  research, 108, 118, 121, 128, 140
  synthesis, 111
Prudden, T. Mitchell, *10, 14*
publications, 49, 66

R
Rasmussen, Howard, *100-101*
Ratliff, Floyd, 85
retroviruses, 102
Rh factor, 72
rheumatic fever, 76
ribonuclease, 108, 111
Rice, Charles, 125
rinderpest
Rivers, Thomas, 76, *76-77*
RNA, 50, 70, 108
  polymerase, *140*
Rockefeller, David, 36, *82-83,* 84, 85, 89, *100-101,* 125, 142-144
Rockefeller, John D., *13, 38*
  financial support for Institute, 7, 15, 16, 22, 25, 26, 34, 125, 142
  Institute founding, 11, 12-13, 15, 142
  Institute visit, 45
  Ledger A, *39*
  philanthropy philosophy, 8, 38
  support for science, 39
Rockefeller, John D., Jr., 13, *13,* 15, 22, *38, 40-41,* 84, 125, 142
Rockefeller Foundation, 26, 28, 39, 41, 49
Rockefeller Hospital, *23, 37, 42-43, 44,* 128, 133
  construction, 34, 42
  clinical research, 25, 52, 105, 106, 124
  Flexner's plan for, 22
  heroin addiction research, 105
  laboratories, 25
  World War II role, 76, *76-77*
Rockefeller Institute for Medical Research, *6, 42-43. See also* Rockefeller University.
  art collection, 89, *90*

boards. *See* Directors, Board of; Scientific Directors, Board of; Trustees, Board of; names of specific members.
budget, 7, 116
building sites, 13, 16, *16,* 17
campus construction, *10, 17,* 42, *42, 82-83,* 86, 89
charter class, 85-86, 100, *100-101*
cultural resources, 8, 86, 89, 117
degree-granting status, 85, 143
faculty and staff. *See* faculty
in fiction, 31
founding, 11-26
Gasser's administration, 75, 83, 84-85
hospital. *See* Rockefeller Hospital.
incorporations, 15, 85
influence, 7, 26, 41, 83
interdisciplinary approach, 56, 86, 92, 143
laboratories. *See* laboratories.
landscape design, 91, *91*
members, 46, 52
mission, 84
as model, 26, 49, 143
name change, 85
Nobel Prizes awarded. *See* Nobel Prize.
publications, 49, 66, 102
research freedom, 8, 13, 19-20, 22, 54, 75, 116
research grants awarded by, 15-16, 32
research leadership, 26, 41, 64, 86
support staff, 45, 46, *46,* 78
university transition, 92, 95
war role, 28, 41, 76, 76-77
women at, *34, 35,* 46, *46-47*
Rockefeller Institute Press, 66
Rockefeller Sanitary Commission, 39
Rockefeller University. *See also* Rockefeller Institute for Medical Research.
  awards, 95, 116. *See also* names of specific awards and prizes.
  budget, 95, 116
  campus, 117
  current research, 116-117
  education programs, 118, 124
  faculty, 95-96, 148-149. *See also* faculty; names of specific faculty members.
  graduate program, 117
  interdisciplinary approach, 117, 118, 121-124, 125, 130
  interinstitutional cooperation, 95-96, 118, 125
  presidents, 97. *See also* names of specific presidents.
  research freedom, 116, 124-125, 130
  restructuring, 8, 95, 96
Rockefeller University Press, 66
Roeder, Robert G., 133, *140-141*
rotating disk viscometer, 78
Rous, Peyton, 7, 28, 49, 102, *103*
Rous sarcoma virus, 60, 102
Rubin, Harry, 102

S
Sabin, Florence, 46
Šali, Andrej, *117*
scarlet fever, 76
Schermerhorn farm, *16, 16*
Scientific Directors, Board of, 64
sea urchin eggs, 51-52
Seitz, Frederick, 95-96, 97, *112-113,* 143
Senate, tenured faculty, 95
set point mechanism, 106
Shannon, James, 84
Shepley, Rutan, and Coolidge (architects), 42
Shih, David, *128-129*
Shope, Richard, 76, 102
Siekevitz, Philip, 62, 118
Simon, Harold J., *100-101*
Smith, Theobald, *14,* 19, 26
Smogorzewska, Agata, *138-139*
solid-phase peptide synthesis, 111
Spelman College, 38, 39
Sputnik satellite, *112-113*
src gene, 102
SREBP-1 protein, 128
Stanley, Wendell M., 26, 70, *70-71*
Starr Center for Human Genetics, 128
Stat3, 133
Stein, William, 75, 108, *108, 109*
Steinman, Ralph M., 134
Stoffel, Markus, 128, *128-129*
streptococcal bacteria, 76
structural biology, 117, 121, 122-123, 140
students, 85-86, 117, 124, 130
Sumner, James B., 70, *70-71*
surgery, 28, *28-29*
Swift, Homer, 45

T
Tatum, Edward, 92
telomeres, 138, *138*
Temin, Howard, 102
Terrell, Edward E., *57*
tissue culture research, 64
tobacco mosaic virus, 70
Tomasz, Alexander, 122
transcription, 133
trypanosomiasis, 34, 35
Tryparsamide, 35
Trustees, Board of, 85
tuberculosis, 11, 122

U
Uhlenbeck, George, 92

V
vaccine, rinderpest, 76
van Breugel, Mark, *138-139*
Van Slyke, Donald D., *21,* 41, 54, *54,* 80, 105, *105*
virology, 26, 70
virus
  cancer cause, 7, 102
  crystallization, 70
  research, 64, 76, 125
vision research, 85

W
War Demonstration Hospital, 28, *28*
Weaver, Warren, 84
Weisner, Jerome B., *112-113*
Weiss, Paul, 92
Welch, William H., *14, 15,* 22, *40-41,* 49, 102, 143
Welch Hall, 42, 46, 68, *68-69,* 86
Wiesel, Torsten N., 85, 96, 97, 98, 143
women, *34, 35,* 46-47, 76, *76*
Woolley, D. Wayne, 41, 111
World War I, 28, 41
World War II, 76, *76-77*
wound treatment, 28

Y
yellow fever, 35, 39
York and Sawyer (architects), 42
Young, Donald A., *100*

Z
Zinder, Norton, 57

153

ILLUSTRATION CREDITS

All illustrations are published courtesy of the Rockefeller Archive Center unless listed below.

Cover: The Rockefeller University Office of Public Affairs

page 6, Yanik Wagner

page 31, Library of Congress reproduction no. LC-USZ62-14119

pages 32-33, © New York City Department of Health, Collection of The New-York Historical Society

page 37, as published in *The New York Architect*, June 1911

page 45, The Rockefeller University Office of Public Affairs

page 58, Ingbert Grüttner

page 66, courtesy The Rockefeller University Press

page 71, UPI/Corbis-Bettmann

page 77, Corbis/Bettman-UPI

page 78, © Barry Dworkin

pages 80-81, © Barry Dworkin

page 82, © The New York Times

page 85, Don C. Young

page 89, © The New York Times

page 91, courtesy The Rockefeller University Office of Plant Operations, with permission from Dan Kiley

page 92, Ingbert Grüttner

page 96, courtesy Patricia Tellerday

page 97, Robert Reichert

page 102, The Rockefeller University Office of Public Affairs

page 104, © Bettmann/Corbis

page 105, The Rockefeller University Office of Public Affairs

page 107, The Rockefeller University Office of Public Affairs

page 110, © Barry Dworkin

page 112, Corbis/Bettman-UPI

page 113, courtesy National Academy of Sciences

page 114, courtesy Gary Schneider and P.P.O.W. Gallery, New York City; specimen prepared by Dorothy Warburton, Columbia Presbyterian Medical Center, New York City

page 117, Arnold Adler

page 119, © Reuters/Anders Wiklund/Archive Photos

page 120, Robert Reichert

page 122, © Huntington Potter, Science Source/Photo Researchers

page 123, courtesy A. James Hudspeth

page 124, The Rockefeller University Office of Public Affairs

page 126, The Rockefeller University Office of Public Affairs

page 128, courtesy Jeffrey Friedman

page 129, Arnold Adler

pages 130-131, Michael Dames

page 132, courtesy Arnold J. Levine

page 133, Dirk Westphal

pages 134-135, courtesy laboratory of Ralph Steinman

page 136, courtesy Roderick MacKinnon

page 137, Robert Reichert

page 138, Arnold Adler

page 139, courtesy Titia de Lange

page 140, courtesy Seth Darst

page 141, Robert Reichert

page 147, courtesy Elizabeth Hanson

This book was designed by Susan Evans, principal of Design per se
in New York City. The typeface used for the narrative text is Stemple Garamond
and the sidebar text is set in Foundry Journal Bold. The book was printed
by The Stinehour Press, Lunenburg, Vermont, and bound by Acme Book Bindery,
Charlestown, Massachusetts, in an edition of 5,000 copies.

About the Author

Elizabeth Hanson is a historian and science writer at
The Rockefeller University. She received her Ph.D. in history and
sociology of science from the University of Pennsylvania.